FEMININE FASTING

THE MOST EFFECTIVE INTERMITTENT FASTING
TRANSFORMATION FOR WOMEN TO LOSE WEIGHT,
RESTORE METABOLISM, AND FINALLY SEE RESULTS!

JOSH COLON

© **Copyright 2022 - All rights reserved.**

The content contained within this book may not be reproduced, duplicated, or transmitted without direct written permission from the author or the publisher.

Under no circumstances will any blame or legal responsibility be held against the publisher, or author, for any damages, reparation, or monetary loss due to the information contained within this book, either directly or indirectly.

Legal Notice:

This book is copyright protected. It is only for personal use. You cannot amend, distribute, sell, use, quote, or paraphrase any part, or the content within this book, without the consent of the author or publisher.

Disclaimer Notice:

Please note the information contained within this document is for educational and entertainment purposes only. All effort has been executed to present accurate, up-to- date, reliable, and complete information. No warranties of any kind are declared or implied. Readers acknowledge that the author is not engaged in rendering legal, financial, medical, or professional advice. The content within this book has been derived from various sources. Please consult a licensed professional before attempting any techniquesoutlined in this book.

By reading this document, the reader agrees that under no circumstances is the author responsible for any direct or indirect losses incurred as a result of the use of the information contained within this document, including, but not limited to, errors, omissions, or inaccuracies.

CONTENTS

Introduction	7
1. WHAT IS FASTING AND WHY SHOULD YOU CARE?	13
What Is Intermittent Fasting?	15
Different Types of Intermittent Fasting	17
What Can I Eat?	20
Is It Safe to Eat this Way?	21
Busting Fasting Myths	23
How Effective Is Intermittent Fasting for Weight Loss?	24
A New Way of Eating	28
2. ADVANTAGES OF INTERMITTENT FASTING FOR WOMEN	31
The Health Risks Linked to Being Overweight	33
The Danger Lurking in Processed Foods	36
The Benefits of Intermittent Fasting	38
3. FASTING AND YOUR HORMONES	49
What Role Do Hormones Play Inside the Human Body?	49
How Does Intermittent Fasting Affect Your Hormones?	51
Is Intermittent Fasting a Safe Option for Women?	54
Can Women Fast During Their Period?	56
Can I Incorporate Intermittent Fasting During Menopause?	57
Tips to Make Intermittent Fasting Easier	59
Why Is Estrogen So Important?	60
More on the Growth Hormone	62

The Impact on Digestive Hormones	64
Intermittent Fasting–A Way to Bring Your Hormones Back into Balance	67

4. BUILDING DISCIPLINE 69
Kickstart Change with the Right Motivation 69
How to Remain Disciplined in Your Intermittent Fasting 71
Tips to Help You Stick to This New Habit 77
Intermittent Fasting and Your Budget 86

5. INTERMITTENT FASTING FOR WOMEN BELOW 30 87
Finding the Best Fasting Schedule 88
Choosing the Best Fasting Foundation 92
Intermittent Fasting and Exercise 92
Tips to Help Make Your Exercise Regime Easy 94
Fasting to Manage Your Weight 96
Fasting for Diabetes 98
Tips for Safe Intermittent Fasting for Type 1 Diabetes Patients 101
Intermittent Fasting and Lasting Youth and Beauty 102

6. INTERMITTENT FASTING FOR WOMEN IN THEIR 30S AND 40S 107
The Most Predominant Changes in Women 30 Years and Older 108
The Benefits of Intermittent Fasting During the 30s and 40s 110
Fasting Tips in Your 30s and 40s 114
Exercise and Intermittent Fasting in Your 30s and 40s 115
The Best Way to Lose Weight Fast 116
Fasting for Diabetes in Your 30s and 40s 120
How Fasting Can Improve Your Mental and Emotional State 122

7. INTERMITTENT FASTING FOR WOMEN 50
   AND OVER   125
   The Benefits of Intermittent Fasting Over 50   127
   Different Types of Intermittent Fasting to
   Consider Beyond Your 50s   129
   Weight Loss Beyond 50   133
   Intermittent Fasting and Diabetes for Women
   Above 50   135
   Fasting to Look Younger   137
   Intermittent Fasting and Medication   139

8. RECIPES   143
   Blueberry Granola Treat   144
   Spicy Dal for a Cold Day   146
   Pizza the Healthy Way   149
   Healthy Burritos   152
   Millet and Quinoa–Tasty and Healthy   154
   Black-Eyed Peas for a Slow Day   157
   Salty and Satisfying Oats Bowl   158
   Bone Broth   161
   A Final Word   165

   Conclusion   167
   Bibliography   169

BEFORE YOU GO ANY FURTHER...

Grab Your Free Book Triple Fasting

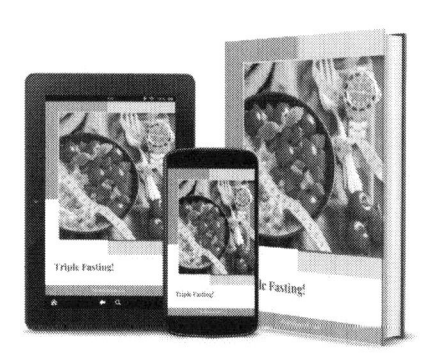

IN HERE YOU WILL LEARN:

3 Key Secrets You **MUST DO** Before Starting Your Intermittent Fasting Journey!

Scan the QR code:

INTRODUCTION

Don't you just hate to see people suffer emotionally, especially if you know that you have knowledge that will help them live a better, happier, and more fulfilled life?

The world of an attorney is fast-paced and stressful. It offers a lifestyle that makes it very hard to sustain balance and follow a healthy diet. I know because my best friend is busy making a name for herself as one of the best up-and-coming criminal lawyers in the city.

My best friend is a girl. She has been my best friend since the day when she came to sit next to me when we were only four or five years old, and she shared her peanut butter and jam sandwich with me. As I am extremely proud of her, I enjoy it when she asks me to accompany her to black-tie events. At some point, these events became more stressful. My friend has such a hectic schedule, so she has been picking up weight over the past two or three years. This is a major problem when she has to get dressed in a formal gown, and her outer appearance just doesn't do justice to who she truly is on a professional and personal level.

It was before such an event that she had a complete meltdown. The week was long and stressful, and she crashed completely when her zipper popped on our way to the function. It was when I knew she desperately needed to hear the dietary advice I had to give her. It was the advice that would help her shed the weight that she had gained so that she could feel better about herself again, be much fitter, and be the best version of herself, for she deserves nothing less.

Do you sometimes wish that you could drop just a few pounds? Maybe it is even more than a few, but you don't know how or where to start or which dietary advice to follow. The more time goes by, the harder it becomes to shed that muffin top sitting so comfortably around your waist. It quickly becomes that one thing you can't miss when you look in the mirror and, after a while, it is all you can see.

As a qualified professional working in the health field, I knew how I could help her. As her friend, I had to convince her to carefully take my advice and guidance regarding her weight concerns.

In my career, I've often noticed that people mostly change their lifestyles to improve their health when they hit rock bottom. This is a place that varies from one person to the next, but for her, rock bottom was the day when her dress popped open. That was three years ago.

While it was a terribly low point for her, it was good, as she was now willing to receive my advice and follow my instructions. She was eager to learn and to change her situation around, and she did. After a year, she has lost 50 lbs and has kept it off. She is healthy, happy, glowing, and, above all, still extremely successful in her career. My best friend has learned how to excel in her professional life without neglecting her body, and one cornerstone of her success has been that she included intermittent fasting as part of her life.

What I am sharing in this book is the same tried and tested advice that I've given her and that brought about so much success in her life. We will touch on exactly what intermittent fasting is and what benefits you can enjoy from making this part of your daily eating habits.

While men and women have hormones, women go through far more hormonal fluctuations in their lives, which affects their health and weight. Intermittent fasting is a wonderful way to take control of your fluctuating hormonal levels before they take control of your life.

For many, the idea of going without food is frightening. As you progress through the book, you'll learn that even initially, it is not as bad as many think. I am also sharing tips on how you can remain disciplined in this way of eating.

As women age, they also undergo several physical changes, which is why we will discuss this type of eating to enjoy exceptional results regardless of whether you are younger than 30 or over the 50 mark. Lastly, I am sharing some recipes to promote your culinary creativity.

During the four years that I was working toward obtaining my degree in biomedical science, the impact of intermittent fasting was a topic we would often discuss in class. We came to realize that fasting is one of the most misunderstood topics. Most people would immediately assume that fasting requires eating nothing for at least 24 hours, preferably longer. This misconception, coupled with many lies that are spread regarding the number of meals you need to eat, what types of foods you need to eat, and what you need to stay away from, contribute to widespread obesity and related health concerns.

While these misconceptions might appear to be innocent, it hurts the lives of those who don't know better and who trust that the advice they get regarding eating is good, while it is not. These are the people who struggle with their weight, have challenges sustaining their overall health and well-being, and pay the price not only physically but also mentally and emotionally.

In my profession, I consider sharing valid and valuable information as my duty. In my personal life, I could see the impact that my advice had on my friend, and I am grateful for being able to instigate such a change. It is why I love to share this information with you, too, hoping that you will experience the same transformation as my friend did.

When we look at the words intermittent fasting, people often scan over 'intermittent' because they are not sure what it entails, and they only hear 'fasting.' It is time that this misconception gets broken by learning the facts about what intermittent fasting is and how it can benefit you.

1

WHAT IS FASTING AND WHY SHOULD YOU CARE?

Everyone who does intermittent fasting talks about it as a lifestyle, not a diet. They come for weight loss but stay for health benefits.

— CELIA SHATZMAN

Benjamin Franklin said that the two best medicines in the world are rest and fasting (Top 25 Fasting Quotes, n.d.). I couldn't agree more. There was a time when both came naturally to humankind, as our lifestyles differed. At ages when food was not readily available, people had to hunt for their food or find berries, fruits, or nuts to eat. These were not always available on-demand, and it would mean that there were times when people had to go without food for extended periods. Getting enough sleep wasn't a problem either, as when darkness fell, there was nothing to do but sleep. They aligned the rhythm of an ordinary day with that of nature.

Today, things are so much different. Food is available in the most processed forms on every corner. We can choose between takeout or feasting on junk food available at any convenience store. Society has smart devices that keep us awake until late at night, and while these screens consume our attention, we snack. While we are working, we snack at our desks. Our bodies hardly ever get the time to cleanse themselves or to use their resources for anything but digestion.

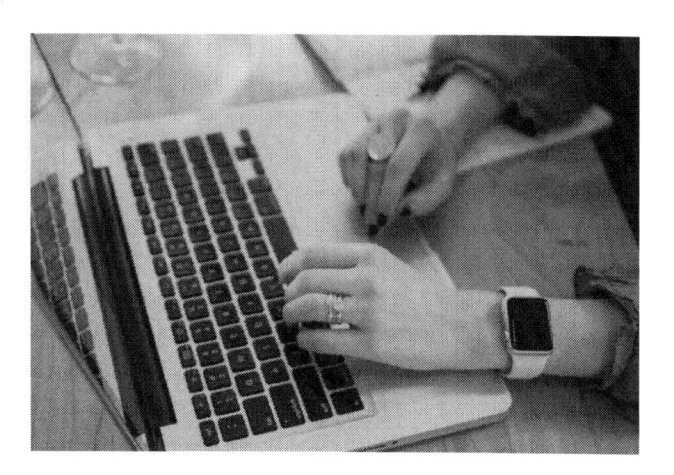

We are walking less, sitting more, and driving to where we need to be. Technology has replaced physical labor, leaving us sitting behind a computer for most of the day. Even when we do attempt to exercise by going for a walk or joining a gym, we don't go without

Making a stop at the snack bar. We exercise with an energy smoothie in our hands. We never take a break from food anymore.

Therefore, it is no wonder that our bodies give in. We develop all kinds of diseases and medical concerns. Diabetes, high blood pressure, high cholesterol levels, various kinds of cancers, heart attacks, and the list goes on. We are a generation that is busy eating ourselves into an early grave.

WHAT IS INTERMITTENT FASTING?

The term fasting refers to a set phase when a person would willfully refrain from eating any food or having any drinks. Traditionally, this is something that often goes along with the religious practice, as many religions would combine fasting with prayer. The term can also refer to the state that our bodies enter when we haven't eaten for some time, often overnight. It is linked to our metabolic state once we have digested all food after a meal.

Intermittent fasting is closely related, but there are several ways in which it differs from fasting. It is mostly a practice followed for health reasons, often to establish weight loss. It also means that there are certain set times when you choose to refrain from food. This period can last for several hours to several days. While you have the choice to involve religion in your intermittent fasting, it is seldom the case, as most people opt to make intermittent fasting a lifestyle choice for the health reasons they can reap from this way of eating.

There are several ways you can choose to include intermittent fasting in your life. By doing so, you access a range of health benefits, and only one of these is that you will lose weight.

Before choosing a specific plan to try out, it is best to understand exactly how intermittent fasting works. While our bodies are still working through the food supply we've consumed, it relies on the sugars and carbs in our meals for instant energy. The body stores all excess energy as fat. When there is never a time when you go without food, your body never reaches a point where it reverts to stored fat for energy. This is especially true if your schedule is so crammed that you never have time to exercise.

By creating food-free windows, you force your body to turn to these food sources and burn the fat that it has stored. While we will discuss the benefits you'll enjoy from intermittent fasting in the next chapter, I feel it is important to mention it here already.

While your body is busy digesting, most of your bodily functions center on the digestive system. It has fewer resources available to take care of cell rejuvenation, combating diseases, and speeding up healing. Once you allow your digestive system time to rest, these other vital tasks happen at a faster pace.

DIFFERENT TYPES OF INTERMITTENT FASTING

Before you jump in, discussing your eating plans with your doctor is always better. These professionals are familiar with your specific medical state and will be able to advise you on what would be the most beneficial solution for you.

The key would be to pick a certain set period that you deliberately go without food. Here you can opt for a daily or a weekly approach.

16/8 Fasting

This is one of the more widely used options, as it is so easy to follow. What it means is that during the 24-hour cycle, you will have 16 hours that you don't eat and eight during which you will consume all the food your body needs. While 16 hours might sound like a long time without food, it is quite easy if you time it around bedtime. Say that you have your last meal around six at night every night, and you don't eat your first meal before ten the next morning. That is 16 hours without food. So, you will eat between 10 a.m. and 6 p.m., which is eight hours. This sounds much easier now, doesn't it? It is why so many people find it easy to switch to this kind of eating. The biggest concern for many upon their introduction to intermittent fasting is that they will always be hungry. While you are sleeping, you won't feel this; therefore, it is perfect timing to fast according to this schedule.

The 5/2 Approach

This approach circles more around how much you would eat than when you would eat. It allows you to eat the way you are used to for five days of the week. You will limit the number of calories you will be consuming for the two remaining days, though. The recommended number of calories to eat on these two days is between 500 and 600

Calories, which you will have in one meal. You can decide which days would be the best for you to take your one-meal days, and these two days don't have to be back-to-back. So, if your schedule is much better on a Tuesday and a Friday, then you can opt to make these the days on which you will have only one meal, but if you want to make it over the weekend, it is also up to you.

Alternate Day Fasting

This type of fasting is much like the more drastic form of the 5/2 approach, as when you are using this method, you will restrict your calorie intake every second day. While more severe than the 5/2 method, you will never fast, and many people find this option more effective yet sustainable.

OMAD

OMAD stands for "one meal a day," and this type of intermittent fasting states you can eat anything you like during one meal per day. For the rest of the time, you would be only drinking fluids that contain zero calories, and this is how you force your body to burn fat for energy.

Short-Term Drastic Forms of Fasting

Within the range of fasting options available, there are three types of fasting that are rather drastic but can be extremely effective. All three forms entail that you only follow them for a short period and use them along with other more sustainable options. These are:

Juice fasting, during which you will only drink freshly squeezed juice from fruit and vegetables with no pulp or additives. Do not continue with this fasting method for over ten days.

Water fasting stipulates that you only drink water during your fasting period. This can be done for a period from between 24 to 72 hours, but not longer.

Dry fasting requires that you have zero intakes of food or water. While being a risky method for certain people, it also brings some benefits.

I will expand on these three fasting options later in the book.

Extended Periods of Fasting

While it's easy to assume that if a little of something is good for you, more of it must be better, that is not the case, according to Dr. Mark Mattson, a neuroscientist at John

Hopkins. He has been researching intermittent fasting and the effect it has on the body for over 25 years, and he states that longer periods of fasting, for example, 24 hours to even 72 hours are not only risky and might be dangerous but are also not as effective. He states that going without food for such long periods can trigger starvation mode in the body, meaning that it will be reluctant to let go of its resources, making it harder to get rid of stubborn fat (John Hopkins Medicine, 2021).

Adjusting to your new way of eating can take up to two weeks. During this time, everyone's body responds differently, and how your body reacts and how hard or easy this transition is will mostly depend on what your normal way of eating looked like before you opted for intermittent fasting. Some people might feel extremely hungry initially and even be rather cranky and difficult to be around others, while for some, this shift is easy. However, once you are through your first two weeks, you will already start to feel the improvement, and it is usually those who make it through this transition phase who tend to stick to the routine, making this their lifestyle.

WHAT CAN I EAT?

When you are shifting into intermittent fasting, it is important to know what you can eat while fasting and what you can indulge in while not fasting.

While you are in your fasting phase, you can only have zero-calorie drinks. This is mainly water and black coffee and tea with no sugar or even sweeteners. While some carbonated drinks contain zero calories, ask yourself if you think this is the best option for you. These drinks are full of artificial ingredients that don't contribute to your health and well-being, and it is much better to avoid having these.

During your non-fasting phase, it might be tempting to indulge in high-calorie foods that are fried or full of sugar. Try to avoid high-calorie treats, especially if the goal that you want to achieve is to lose weight. Rather stick to foods that are healthy and high in nutrients but lower in calories. Rather than making food the focal point while eating,

make the social experience of eating and spending time with loved ones the core of your meals. When eating, do so mindfully. Focus on what you are eating, what the food tastes like, and what the textures are like that you are enjoying. Take your time to note everything you put into your mouth and chew slowly, as this will not only make you enjoy your food more but also aid in feeling full sooner.

IS IT SAFE TO EAT THIS WAY?

Intermittent fasting works so well to treat a range of medical concerns, including dietary challenges such as irritable bowel syndrome or celiac disease, or even diabetes, cholesterol concerns, and arthritis, but it is not a solution that is available to all.

Those who are better off staying away from this type of eating are children who are still growing, mainly youngsters below the age of 18, women who are pregnant or breastfeeding, and those who have had eating disorders in the past. When you are struggling with blood sugar problems, you must discuss your plans with your medical practitioner first before constricting your food intake in this manner. Also, be careful when you are using chronic medications, have low blood pressure, or are underweight already. Lastly, women who are trying to get pregnant or have had amenorrhea in the past shouldn't start with intermittent fasting unless they speak to a medical professional first.

However, unless you fall into these categories, it is completely safe to transition to intermittent fasting, as it is a way of eating to which the human body adapts easily.

Signs that you need to look out for are when you are experiencing nausea, headaches, anxiety, or any other symptoms you didn't have before your intermittent fasting. While these might result from a detox process that your body could go through, it is best to keep your medical practitioner in the loop to ensure that you remain on a healthy track.

BUSTING FASTING MYTHS

As with anything else in life, there are also several myths surrounding the concept of intermittent fasting. One of the most common myths is that you experience muscle loss if you eat in this manner. This is not completely false, but the entire picture is that you.

will experience muscle loss with any type of dietary restrictions that you follow to lose weight. However, it is proven that with intermittent fasting, the percentage of muscle loss that you'll experience is far less than with other types of dieting. The best way to combat this is to include enough protein in your diet and to build your muscle through regular exercise.

This also busts the next myth, which is that you can't work out when you've opted for intermittent fasting. Not only is exercising perfectly fine, but experts in the field also recommend it as part of a balanced and healthy lifestyle.

Another myth we need to address is that intermittent fasting will slow down your metabolism. This is only a concern when you are fasting for longer periods, but not at all when you opt for shorter periods like with the 16/8 or 5:2 approach. When you rely on either of these options, you will increase the speed of your metabolism.

Lastly, there is a concern that you can't take supplements when fasting. You can continue taking the supplements that you are used to taking. If you are taking a supplement that contains fat-soluble vitamins like vitamins A, D, E, and K, you will enjoy a more effective uptake of these supplements when you take them with your meals.

HOW EFFECTIVE IS INTERMITTENT FASTING FOR WEIGHT LOSS?

While I can easily confirm that intermittent fasting not only works extremely well to establish weight loss, but also that it is a healthy lifestyle that is highly beneficial if you want to improve your overall well-being, you don't have to take my word for it. Except for my best friend, whose story I already mentioned in the introduction, there are many other women just like you who have enjoyed immense weight loss simply by changing when they eat rather than what they eat. I am sharing some of these success stories with you.

Melissa Bunch

Between June 2021 and March 2022, Melissa lost 100 lbs. She shed all this weight in a mere ten months simply by opting for intermittent fasting. Melissa shared she was always eating. It didn't matter what she was busy with; she would nibble on something. While constantly eating, though, she considered herself to be a rather healthy eater and

would opt for healthy options to snack on. Thus, the problem that led to Melissa's yo- yoing that stretched over three decades wasn't that she indulged in unhealthy food.

She just never gave her body a break from eating. The primary concern of her body remained to digest the constant supply of food it had to deal with, and not only did this cause her to be overweight, but it also brought about a range of other health concerns.

It was only when her blood pressure became so bad that she suffered a mini-stroke at 41, that she hit rock bottom and knew that she had to do something that would bring her the results she desired. Not only were her kids still very little, but she also had a son with Down syndrome who needed his mom to be around.

Within a few months of starting with intermittent dieting, Melissa's blood pressure returned to normal, and she continuously shed weight every month. She states she realized that every day she had a choice to make, to be responsible by being disciplined in the way she was eating or to fall back into her old routines. Yet, as she was not only losing weight but also feeling healthy and strong, she became more positive and energetic. She kept her weight off instead of gaining it all back again, as it had happened so often for her in the past. Melissa states she is now living a new life, and food is no longer the thing that consumes her thoughts all the time (Success Stories, n.d.).

Dana McMahan

For Dana McMahan, intermittent fasting happened by accident, but it is an accident she is very glad happened to her.

While Dana wasn't dealing with a lot of weight that she had to shed, it was stubborn weight, and she struggled to drop the extra pounds. Then the pandemic hit the globe, and everyone was in a state of stress. While some people turn to food during stressful times (one of the main reasons so many people gained weight during this period of isolation), Dana lost her appetite. She found that she hardly ever ate breakfast anymore, as she was so stressed all the time. While this initially concerned her, she later learned that breakfast was a relatively recent addition to the eating habits of people. Humans haven't always been eating three meals a day.

As she isn't someone who would often find herself on the scale, she initially didn't notice that she was losing weight, and it was only when she realized her clothes were fitting much looser that she realized she was shedding her extra pounds. The idea of intermittent fasting became interesting to her as she noticed the success she was enjoying, and she opted to study it in greater detail and made this a lifestyle choice for her. In total, Dana lost 20 lbs and is feeling energized and amazing (MacMahan, 2020).

Martine Etienne-Mesubi

It might be all well and good to tell anyone who is struggling to shed the extra weight that they need to follow a healthy diet and be more active. However, this is not the lifestyle that is enjoyed or even practical for all. Martine is one of the people for whom the latter is true.

She didn't enjoy being on a diet, and exercise wasn't a favored activity either, but she knew she had to do something as she was 42 years old and weighed 225 lbs. She couldn't run and play with her 6-year-old daughter, and she even had to stop at times to catch herbreath when the two of them walked to the park.

It was when her second daughter was born that she lost any structure in her eating habits, having a meal late at night and then going to bed sleeping on a full tummy. An added concern in the mind of this mother was that both diabetes and high blood pressure were medical concerns that were quite common in her family. She knew she couldn't get sick as her children needed her.

Martine researched intermittent fasting and tried several ways of fasting to see which worked the best for her. She also realized that when she became hungry, she only had to drink something like tea or water and shift her focus to something else, and the hunger would pass.

Martine lost 80 lbs by sticking to intermittent fasting. She reduced her eating window to only one meal per day which she would have with her family. She states that when it is holiday time, she reverts to a 6-8 hour eating window, but once they are back in their routine, she is back to having only one meal a day (OMAD).

Martine states that not only is she feeling healthy and happy but also confident in her body, and it is this boost in her self-esteem that is truly bringing about the success that she is now enjoying in her career (Thurrott, 2020).

Sarah Walton Steele

The older women get, the harder it can be for them to shed the extra weight. As we age, this additional weight easily becomes a much greater health risk too. Thus, the story of the 64-year-old Sarah is truly inspirational. Sarah weighed 242 lbs and was only 5'3". She has been struggling with her weight all her life and has been on many diets that would help her lose weight, and then she would only pick it all up again.

In a matter of nine months, Sarah lost 50 lbs simply by opting for OMAD as her preferred way of intermittent fasting. Sarah states that she doesn't deny herself any food and eats whatever she feels like, but she restricts when she eats. She states that she even has dessert every day and still maintains her weight loss. She describes this way of eating as her new lifestyle and states that it is something that she enjoys.

A NEW WAY OF EATING

I started this chapter with a quote by Benjamin Franklin about rest and fasting. Both of these used to be part of the way humans lived. Then a range of advances came about, changing the world in so many ways that also affected the way we sleep and eat. Over recent years, studies have highlighted the importance of getting enough sleep, and now we are far more aware of how vital it is to get the right number of hours of sound sleep every night.

What we are also now witnessing is that more people are noticing the fact that intermittent fasting is vital to enjoy and sustain good overall health. More people are moving back to a way of eating where they eat fewer meals during the day and cut back on snacking in between meals.

We also realize that breakfast hasn't always been part of our daily routine and that it means breaking your fast. Until recently, only a few people opted for this kind of eating, but far more are doing it now, and we can only hope that this healthy practice will return as a mainstream way of eating to combat the immensely negative impact that modern- day living has on our eating habits and our well-being.

2

ADVANTAGES OF INTERMITTENT FASTING FOR WOMEN

To eat is a necessity but to eat intelligently is an art.

— FRANÇOIS DE LA ROCHEFOUCAULD

There is probably no simple explanation as to why living a healthy lifestyle is more important than what Jim Rohn captured when he stated that we need to "Take care of your body. It's the only place you have to live." (Rohn, n.d.)

I want to circle back to hitting rock bottom. When thinking about hitting rock bottom in our lives, two questions come to mind. The first is why we so often need to hit rock bottom before we make the much-needed changes in our lives, and the other is, what does rock bottom look like?

Let me start by answering the first question. Often, we are completely aware of the fact that we need to change our habits, but we just don't. This is because change is uncomfortable, and nobody likes to step out of their comfort zones unless it becomes necessary. Rock bottom is often that moment when it becomes necessary when the alternative is not something we can live with. Maybe the alternative is too painful, too dangerous, or simply life-threatening. It is why you'll see that it is often only once the doctor gives people bad news about their health that they will do something about it, making smarter choices in their diet and becoming more active. It is not just the case with our physical health but also in our relationships, our careers, and more. Thus, maybe you are keen on making the much-needed changes because you've received bad news regarding your own health.

The second question is harder to answer. How do you know that you've reached rock bottom? This is a personal question that varies from one person to the next. While someone suffering from diabetes is completely fine with the idea that they will have to inject themselves daily to survive, someone else might consider the idea of having to do that as hitting rock bottom.

You will know when you can't continue like you have been doing for probably a very long time.

What I can share with you before we delve into the many benefits that you can enjoy from intermittent fasting are the many health risks that you will face (if you aren't already) if you don't drop the added weight that you are carrying around. These are also factors that affect not only your physical well-being but also your mental and emotional states.

THE HEALTH RISKS LINKED TO BEING OVERWEIGHT

I do not intend this segment to scare you, but sadly, it is the reality that everyone will have to face at a certain point in their lives if they don't take care of themselves and make their physical health a priority in their lives. This list only covers the most commonly associated health risks linked to being overweight.

Type 2 Diabetes

Maybe you are aware of the fact that there are two types of diabetes. The one that is linked to being overweight is type 2 diabetes, which is prevalent in people who have a blood sugar level that is above normal. If this is a medical health concern that runs in your family, you are at an even greater risk of getting this type of diabetes (National Institute of Diabetes and Digestive and Kidney Diseases, 2019). While we can manage diabetes, it leads to various more serious health concerns like kidney disease, nerve damage, strokes, and heart disease. People who are suffering from diabetes also often have poor blood circulation, which causes slow healing of wounds.

High Blood Pressure

The simplest explanation of high blood pressure is that the force of the blood in your veins is higher than normal, and this puts added stress on the vein walls and your organs, especially your heart. The result is that you are at greater risk of stroke or heart attack, but it can also damage your kidneys. These concerns can be fatal.

Heart Attacks and Strokes

We have partially covered both in the previous two paragraphs. Heart attacks are far more prevalent in those who have high blood pressure, high blood sugar, or high cholesterol levels.

A stroke occurs when one of your artery walls bursts because of the pressure it's under from having consistently high blood pressure levels. This causes damage to the

surrounding tissue and can reduce the blood supply to vital organs, such as your brain specifically.

Sleep Apnea

Sleep apnea refers to a condition where you stop breathing while you are sleeping. It is a concern that is far more common in people who are overweight, and what normally happens is that your body gets deprived of oxygen, and usually, the person would gasp for air, waking themselves up. This exposes your body to even greater tension, and it robs you of good quality sleep.

Fatty Liver Disease

This disease results from a build-up of fat in the liver tissue, and it causes various other liver concerns, such as cirrhosis, liver damage, and liver failure.

Gallbladder Disease

The gall bladder and the liver are closely linked to each other. When you are overweight, and your liver is under pressure, you are more likely to develop gallstones.

Kidney Diseases

The kidney is another organ that is closely linked to the liver and the gallbladder. When you have high blood pressure or blood sugar levels, your kidneys are likely under strain to filter your blood. Being under too much strain for too long causes weaknesses in the kidney that can snowball into kidney failure.

Challenges to Conceive

Ladies who are overweight are likely to struggle more than those who are not to fall pregnant. When they fall pregnant, they are also exposing themselves far more to various concerns, and they are facing far more challenges during the pregnancy.

Various Cancers

Several types of cancers are far more prevalent in people who are struggling with their weight.

In these medical concerns, prevention is far better than cure. You have only one body. Make yourself a priority in your life and put your health first.

THE DANGER LURKING IN PROCESSED FOODS

Food has never been as easily available as it is in the modern-day. When you walk down the streets in your city, it is more than likely that you can purchase some type of food along your walk from at least one place in the street.

While having access to an abundance of food is not a bad thing, the concern comes in with the food we have access to and not having to exert ourselves in any way to get these foods. I am referring to processed foods. These are foods that are unrecognizably processed and filled with all kinds of chemicals, such as preservatives and flavorings. These foods are high in calories and almost completely robbed of nutrients. The most commonly eaten types of processed foods are:

- Cereals
- Chips
- Crackers
- Candy

- Ready meals
- Instant meals like instant noodles
- Sodas and soft drinks
- Meats that have been processed like nuggets and sausages.

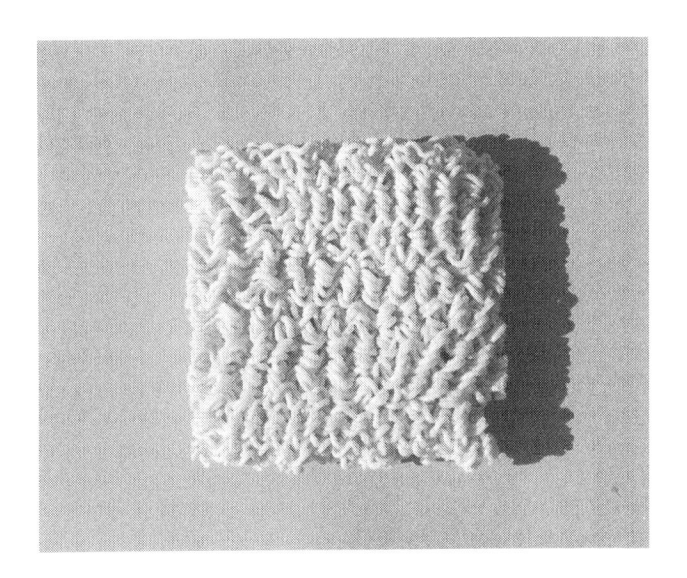

The risk with this kind of food is not only that it is high in calories while providing our bodies with almost no nutrients, but also that, as it is so easy and tasty, we include far too much of this food in our regular diet.

How many servings of this kind of food do you eat per week?

Through a research study that included 20,000 adults, the researcher determined that eating four or more portions of processed foods per week increases your risk of all diseases that can lead to premature death. For every portion that you eat more than the four they've tested, you increase your risk of death by 18% (Pratt, 2020).

These foods are high in sugar and salt content. Processed foods are often fried and thus high in fats, and as they contain very little fiber (if any), they don't leave you feeling full. So, you consume far more than a mere portion.

I am sharing this information regarding processed foods with you because I want you to enjoy the level of success that you deserve. You can achieve amazing results with intermittent fasting, but there is a trap that exists, and I've seen many people step right into it. This trap is the belief that as you are only eating at certain times, you can eat whatever you want during these times. While this is true, it is also not good for you to indulge in processed foods during these times.

You don't have to count every calorie you consume during your eating windows, but please make smart food choices. Eat foods that are healthy and filling and will provide your body with the nutrients and goodness it needs.

Be kind to yourself and eat good food.

THE BENEFITS OF INTERMITTENT FASTING

Now that we've explored the one side of the spectrum, it is time to flip the coin and see what benefits you can enjoy when you follow a lifestyle that includes intermittent fasting.

Weight Loss

Yes, you will enjoy weight loss when you give your body a break from digestion regularly, but what I haven't pointed out yet is that you will also lose visceral fat. Visceral is belly fat, and it is dangerous. On the outside, it presents itself as that tube that you have around your waistline, but on the inside of your body, this is the fat that has wrapped itself around your vital organs. This fat affects your abdominal activity and can cause several concerns. It is also the kind of fat that is often much more challenging to lose.

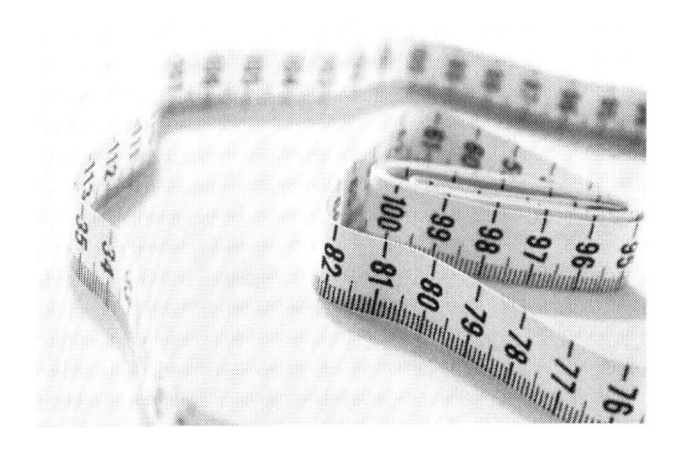

Intermittent fasting works to achieve a weight loss of this magnitude in two ways. One is that you will automatically consume fewer calories as you will eat less. The second way it operates is by supporting better hormone functioning. As there will be more times when your body is not digesting food, you will have lower insulin levels that will lead to higher Human Growth Hormone (HGH) levels that increase the noradrenaline in your blood

which speeds up the breakdown of fat to use this stored energy. Therefore, studies showed that people who fast intermittently could lose between 3-8% of their body weight over a period from as little as three weeks to 24 weeks (Gunnars, 2016).

Less Likely to Develop Type 2 Diabetes

I don't want to expend too much on this again, but the people who follow intermittent fasting are far less likely to develop type 2 diabetes. This is mostly because they are less likely to develop insulin resistance.

Intermittent Fasting Improves Hormonal Function

When we eat, various hormonal changes occur in the body. When we fast, these functions change. The hormones that are most affected by intermittent fasting are:

Insulin levels are lower, and this increases your body's ability to burn fat for energy.

The level of HGH in your body increases, and this contributes to fat burning but also muscle gain, combatting the loss of muscle mass that often goes along with weight loss.

However, changes not only take place on a hormonal level but also on a cellular level.

It becomes easier for the body to get rid of the waste that gathers inside the cells of your body, and this process speeds up cell repair.

Lastly, it contributes to gene expression, so it brings about changes in genes that contribute to longevity and protection against diseases.

Minimize Inflammation

When we look at many of the well-known chronic diseases, we notice that these are often the result of high levels of oxidative stress that we expose our bodies to. Oxidative stress results from the number of free radicals that can be found inside your cells. When free radicals attach themselves to the DNA in your body, they damage the cells.

Several studies have shown that intermittent fasting aids in the body's ability to protect itself against oxidative stress. Not only does this slow down aging, but it also prevents inflammation in the body tissue (Gunnars, 2016).

Speed Up Cellular Repair

Intermittent fasting is not only an excellent way of reducing the level of inflammation in your body, but it also contributes to speeding up cell repair. Cellular repair occurs when your body breaks down damaged or broken cells and replaces them with new ones. Ensuring that your cellular repair is taking place at an optimal speed reduces your chances of various dreaded diseases like cancer and Alzheimer's disease.

Prevent Various Forms of Cancer

Cancer results from uncontrolled cell growth. Some of the more recent test-tube studies indicated that periods of fasting are as effective in slowing down the growth of tumors as chemotherapy (Link, 2018). While much work still needs to be done to see if intermittent fasting can be a viable and effective treatment for cancer, the results appear promising.

Improves Heart Health

As heart disease is a major health concern with a global impact, many studies have determined the most predominant risk factors for heart disease and failure. Some risks that researchers have identified are high blood sugar, blood pressure, and cholesterol levels. Another concern that is often far less spoken about is high levels of inflammation. If your body is in a constant state of inflammation, the odds of developing heart disease are much higher. As these concerns are reduced when you opt to do intermittent fasting, it can significantly reduce your chances of getting heart disease.

Improved Brain Health

How does the way we eat impact our brain health? Quite simply, it provides the brain with the same benefits that all the other cells in your body enjoy from having better control over your hormonal levels. Intermittent fasting supports brain health by reducing inflammation and controlling your blood sugar levels. As several studies also show that it increases the growth of nerve cells, it can play a contributing role in preventing several medical concerns.

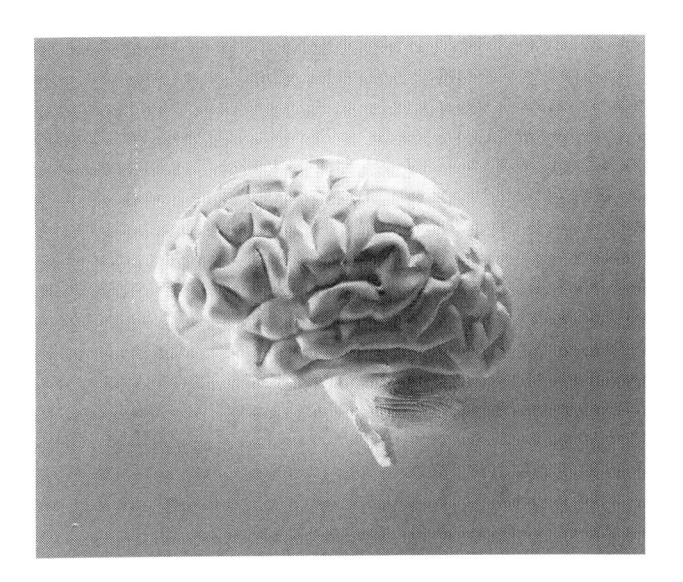

Therefore, there has been a growing interest in how intermittent fasting can help to reduce the symptoms of Alzheimer's disease. Unfortunately, until today, there has been no cure for Alzheimer's disease, and this makes it even more vital that intermittent fasting is explored more to see how medical professionals can optimally use this way of eating to reduce the debilitating impact of the dreaded disease.

The link between intermittent fasting and other brain-related concerns, like Parkinson's disease and Huntington's disease, is also being explored by researchers globally.

There have also been several studies that indicate that intermittent fasting increases the levels of the hormone "brain-derived neurotrophic factor," or BDNF. Medical professionals often associate lower levels of BDNF with patients suffering from depression (Gunnars, 2016). Thus, does not only intermittent fasting improve the physical state of your brain but also the mental state that you are in.

Except for these serious health concerns, you will also be able to enjoy much greater focus. When your body is constantly exposed to food and immersed in the digestive process, it is the case that your blood sugar levels are constantly increasing and dropping, and this leads to feeling lethargic and having difficulty focusing. Are you familiar with that laziness that comes over you after you have a sugar-rich lunch and have to return to your desk? It can feel impossible to focus on the task at hand. When your body goes through fasting phases, you burn fat rather than sugars, as your energy source and fat are, in general, a cleaner form of energy and provides you with a stable supply. Thus, you will miss out on that tiredness that makes it so hard to focus.

Longevity

If I tell you that following a lifestyle that includes intermittent fasting will expand your life, will this convince you to at least try the solution to see how it benefits you? For as long as humankind has existed, longevity has been something we've been searching for. While intermittent fasting will most likely not provide you with eternal youth, several studies indicate the many ways this way of eating improves your overall well-being and contributes to longevity.

Cell rejuvenation, fewer inflammation markers, and increased metabolism are all factors that should provide you with much better health. Several research studies have already found that daily fasting in mice increases their life span by as much as 13%, while the rats in another study show an increase of 83% in their life span when they are subjected to regular fasting (Gunnars, 2016).

Suffering from Fewer Cravings

Do you often find yourself in a position where you simply want to eat the entire time? Cravings can sometimes be terrible. The more we give in to these cravings, the more we experience them. Cravings result from fluctuations in our blood sugar levels, and when you gain better control over these levels, as one does when you opt for intermittent fasting, these cravings will leave you too.

An Improved Appearance

When was the last time that you had glowing and radiant skin? It might feel that looking older is just something you need to settle for in life. Maybe you are paying exorbitant amounts of money on treatments to regain your youthful appearance. As intermittent fasting speeds up the process of cell rejuvenation, you can be sure to generate new skin cells at a faster pace, too, leaving your skin looking healthy.

Increased Confidence

You will lose weight and look much better by opting for intermittent fasting. The result is that you will feel much better about yourself. You will find that your confidence is growing, and your self-esteem is improving. You might also start to feel that you can take on challenges that you wouldn't have done otherwise. However, intermittent fasting requires discipline, and by holding yourself to this discipline, you will find that you can achieve much more than you might have expected. Often this success helps motivate you to achieve other successes, too.

Feeling Sexy

When was the last time you looked in the mirror, and the word 'sexy' was the first that came to mind? Maybe it has been such a long time that you can't even remember, or maybe it is not a way that you've ever thought about yourself. Every woman has something that makes her sexy. Yes, the sex appeal of some people is very obvious, while others have a more hidden kind of sex appeal that makes them alluring, but the one thing that makes any woman sexy above all others is the way she feels about herself. This affects how you carry yourself and how you present yourself in conversations.

Feeling sexy is not something that you should just dismiss as nothing. On the contrary, it is a factor that influences your overall joy in life, the level of success you'll enjoy in your career, and, asa result thereof, even your financial well-being.

You can be the best version of yourself, regardless of what age you are.

Maybe you are not facing any serious health concerns or aren't constantly tired. Maybe the struggle with your weight has not been taunting you your entire life. These things can be true for you, and still, you might not feel your best. You might not wake up feeling energized or optimistic about the day ahead. If this describes you, don't you think it is time to change to live the best life you possibly can? We only have one life; make it count and live it fully by being in the best state you can be, emotionally, mentally, and physically. Take control of your life. You are an empowered woman, so live like one.

In the next chapter, we are going to explore the role of intermittent fasting and hormones. Hormonal fluctuations play a much more influential role in women's overall well-being, affecting their physical, mental, and emotional states. Thus, let's see how you can take control of your hormones by choosing when you are eating and when you refrain from having any food.

3

FASTING AND YOUR HORMONES

Even a woman of abnormal will cannot escape her hormonal identity.

— CAMILLE PAGLIA

WHAT ROLE DO HORMONES PLAY INSIDE THE HUMAN BODY?

The human body comprises a complex and intricate number of systems that all have to work well together to ensure that you can live life to the fullest. There are many types of hormones present in the body. They fulfill multiple functions:

- Hormones are responsible for growth and development. While this takes place mostly during the teenage years, at a more mature age, hormones contribute to cell renewal and thus ensure healing and prevent premature aging.
- Hormones also control fertility and sexual drive.
- The speed of your metabolism is at an optimal level when your hormonal levels are in a healthy and balanced state.
- Mood swings and increased stress are both aspects that you can gain control over when you have control of your hormones.
- Even body temperature is controlled by your hormones.
- Your hormones play an active role in almost every bodily function that takes place.

When your hormones are out of balance, the following are all health concerns that can present themselves:

- Sudden mood changes
- Increased irritation and even anxiety
- Feeling bloated
- Reduced sex drive
- Dry skin
- Hair that is going dull and is thinning
- Bones go brittle, increasing your chances of breaking something

- Blurred or poor vision
- Increasing heart rate
- Poor sleep and waking up regularly
- Increased thirst
- Problems with your digestive system

As hormones play an important role in our overall well-being, it is important to see how intermittent fasting affects your body, what concerns it can improve, and how this new way of eating will affect men and women differently.

HOW DOES INTERMITTENT FASTING AFFECT YOUR HORMONES?

During the average life cycle, women go through far more hormonal fluctuations than men ever do. First, there is the tremendous impact of an elevation in hormonal levels during the teenage years and adolescence. Men and women go through this change, but then there is also the impact of hormone changes during the monthly cycle for women, pregnancy, and later on, menopause. Thus, women must understand how intermittent fasting can affect their hormones and how it can benefit them when they persist and make this way of eating a life choice. I would also like to address the commonly asked questions of whether intermittent fasting is safe for women in this chapter.

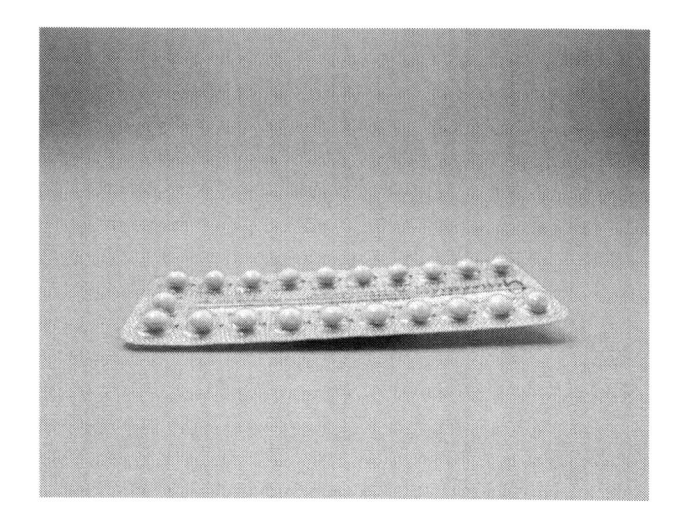

When we look at the impact of intermittent fasting on men and women, it is important to note that men and women react to intermittent fasting in the same manner in many ways and completely different in others.

During a study that took place at the University of Illinois, nutrition professor Kristina Varady determined that men and women show very similar results in terms of weight loss instigated by intermittent fasting. Varady explored the impact of specific time- restricted fasting (16/8) and alternate-day fasting (the 5:2 model) (Putka, n.d.).

Varady also found that their weight and body composition changes were very similar. Both genders showed a slight decrease in their bad cholesterol counts. However,

she found some differences in how premenopausal and postmenopausal women reacted, and she realized a possible link between these differences and the decrease in their bad cholesterol levels (Putka, n.d.).

In another research study, the focal point was to determine the impact of intermittent fasting on glucose response rates in men and women. This study found that women's glucose response rates were slightly worse than that of men and that men had a worse insulin response rate than women after intermittent fasting for several weeks.

There is also evidence that during this kind of fasting, the triglycerides of men accumulate in their livers, and in women, this accumulation takes place in their muscles. Triglycerides are commonly found in natural fats and oils (Putka, n.d.).

While these studies also reported that women indicated they would get hungry more often than their male counterparts did, the difference between the response in the male body when exposed to intermittent fasting and the female body wasn't all that different.

However, something else that resulted as a spin-off from these studies was a deeper discussion regarding why intermittent fasting and the keto way of eating are so closely linked to each other. This is mainly because when the body is in a state of fasting, it shifts from using glucose present in the bloodstream as an energy source to using stored fats as the primary energy resource. This is the same effect that those who are following the ketogenic diet have. When you follow the ketogenic way of eating, you force the body into a state of ketosis. During this phase, the body relies on the ketones created from body fat to provide its fuel. Thus, in both instances, the body uses stored energy, or fat, as an energy source instead of using the glucose present from the constant consumption of sugar and carb-rich foods.

IS INTERMITTENT FASTING A SAFE OPTION FOR WOMEN?

Now that we are aware of the minor differences in the ways the bodies of men and women respond to intermittent fasting, and we operate from the foundation that hormones play a crucial role in the physical and emotional wellness of women, we need to ask, how safe is intermittent fasting for women?

The first determining factor influencing how safe intermittent fasting is for the female body is how much stress your body is already being exposed to. Here, it is important to take note that stress refers not only to stress caused by outside factors such as work conditions, long hours, and pressing deadlines but also to the changes you make to your

lifestyle. However, it is important to realize that some causes of stress can be good for you. These positive sources of stress can include adding exercise to your daily routine and eating in healthier ways, including intermittent fasting.

Therefore, make sure that you manage these changes, and then the stress you'll experience from opting for intermittent fasting will be good for you.

While I am stating this, I also want to highlight that no two bodies are the same or react to things in the same manner. Therefore, I want to emphasize that it is always best to keep track of how your body is behaving when you introduce something new to your habits. While something might work well for someone else, it is not necessarily going to have the same impact on you. So, while the vast majority of women enjoy excellent results from their transition to intermittent fasting, you can't just assume the outcome will be the same for you. It is why we need to explore on a deeper level how and if intermittent fasting can impact and improve your hormonal balance.

Now, let's circle back to the initial question of whether intermittent fasting is safe for women. The female body produces large volumes of a protein called kisspeptin, which plays a vital role in reproduction. This specific hormone is sensitive to factors such as stress.

When the female body releases kisspeptin, it activates another hormone, the gonadotropin-releasing hormone (GnRH). This hormone plays an important role in a much larger chain reaction. GnRH stimulates the production and release of follicle- stimulating hormone (FSH) and luteinizing hormone (LH) in the pituitary gland. These are important as LH stimulates the ovaries to produce estradiol, a form of estrogen and progesterone, and it also stimulates the ovaries to release an egg during ovulation, which is crucial in the reproductive system.

There have been studies that have found that intermittent fasting can reduce the production of kisspeptin, which will have a ripple effect, and this can bring about a complete imbalance in the hormonal levels of the female body. Until this point, these studies were all just performed on animals and not humans. Therefore, while there might be rumors that intermittent fasting can reduce women's chances of falling pregnant, it is important to take note that there are no studies that prove these claims as yet.

Another concern that some might have is that when women fast, their bodies might go into starvation mode, and this will reduce their fertility. However, this might only be the case during long fasting periods and is not the case with intermittent fasting, which appears to have the opposite effect on fertility in women.

CAN WOMEN FAST DURING THEIR PERIOD?

This is one question I get asked the most. During this stage in the female cycle, women feel bloated and more emotional and often indulge in comfort foods. Thus, many women wonder if it is fine to put their bodies through the strain of intermittent fasting, even during this time.

The short answer to this is that it is perfectly fine, but I would like to back this up with the research of Dr. Amy Shah, a double-board-certified physician. She states that the most stressful week for women is not the one when they have their period but the week prior. It is during this week that the female body is most prone to be under stress, as they have lower estrogen levels and a higher sensitivity to cortisol. Cortisol is, of course, the body's stress hormone, and intermittent fasting can increase stress in the lives of women during this time. Thus, if you are fasting and are following the 16:8 schedule, you can consider increasing your eating window to 12 hours instead of eight and reduce the stress that your body experiences. When you reach day zero of your cycle, you can be restrictive again for the next 14 days (Boyers, 2020). While giving this advice, I also want to state that if you are mindful of your eating and are familiar with your body and can quickly gather if something is not the way it should be, you can follow your biological rhythm. Get to know your body and be mindful of it, and your body will guide you to when you have to give yourself a little slack and eat during a larger window and when you are fine to continue with your intermittent fasting.

CAN I INCORPORATE INTERMITTENT FASTING DURING MENOPAUSE?

The time of menopause is the other time in a woman's life when they experience major hormonal changes. The only other time is, of course, pregnancy, a time during which I do not advise intermittent fasting at all. So, is it safe for a woman experiencing menopause to opt for intermittent fasting?

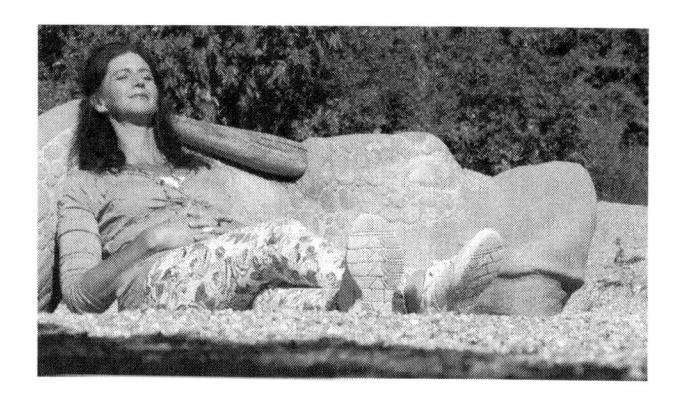

First, let's look at the most predominant changes that take place during this phase. The body of a woman who is approaching her fifties, or is already in her early fifties, can experience a drop in estrogen and progesterone levels. Women during this stage also become less sensitive to the hormone insulin. This may cause slower metabolism, which can, in turn, cause an increase in weight and other changes such as mood swings, feeling foggier and more frequently tired, and increased psychological stress. According to the board-certified doctor and expert in hormonal balance and women's health, Dr. Taz Bhatia, intermittent fasting is not only safe for women in menopause but is also a way to relieve many of the symptoms that go along with this phase in their lives (Boyers, 2020).

During this time, women can experience challenges like lowered self-esteem, the need to feel achievement in their lives, brain stress, and even a degree of depression. These are all symptoms that intermittent fasting can address and improve.

TIPS TO MAKE INTERMITTENT FASTING EASIER

If you are ready to try intermittent fasting but are concerned about how it will affect your life and your hormones, then there are a few tips that will help make the process a bit easier for your body to get used to.

Try to do it only for a few days a week. This will ease your body into a new way of eating. It is often the abruptness of diets that makes them more stressful. So, rather than making an instant switch, opt to ease into it and maybe start with only two days during the week and gradually increase the number of days when you follow the 16/8 way of eating, for example.

If you are already following a strenuous fitness regime, consider taking it a little slower on the days you are fasting and avoid high-intensity training during these days.

While you might have the urge to indulge in various calorie-rich foods, rather opt for foods that have a higher nutrient value, as this will provide your body with what it needs to remain strong and healthy even if you are eating only within certain windows.

However, the best advice remains to listen to your body. If you feel weak during the day, listen to your body instead of sticking rigidly to a set plan. If you are struggling with this, keep a journal and track how your body is feeling. This will give you an indication of what your body is trying to tell you.

Always remember that your body is amazing and unique, and simply taking notice of what you are feeling and experiencing your body will guide you toward the best solution for you.

WHY IS ESTROGEN SO IMPORTANT?

I have said a lot about estrogen levels. I wanted to touch on the role that this hormone fulfills, especially in the female body.

In short, estrogen makes women so different from men. It is the hormone that gives women curves and a softer body. Wider hips and the development of breasts are both influenced by estrogen levels. It plays not only a role in the outer appearance, but it is also an important role player in the biological changes taking place internally. Estrogen helps women to fall pregnant, to have their menstrual cycle, and to have strong bones and beautiful and full hair. On the emotional side, estrogen takes control of a woman's mood and helps with brain development.

When estrogen levels drop to the point of being too low, various concerns can arise. Brittle bones are a major health concern for women who are past fifty and have already experienced menopause. When your estrogen levels have dropped significantly over some time, this can lead to broken bones and causes broken hips when elderly women fall.

Low estrogen levels also cause vaginal dryness, which can cause painful intercourse. Another cause of painful intercourse is thinning vaginal walls.

Weight gain is another outcome when estrogen levels are too low, as the regulation of the body's fat resources becomes less effective and the body stores more fat.

One of the most typical signs of menopause is hot flashes. This is because of the body not being able to regulate its temperature as well anymore.

Women with a lower estrogen level can struggle to fall asleep, wake up more often during the night, and feel tired more often.

These changes also come along with an increase in emotional unease and depression. Having estrogen levels that are too high is also not healthy.

One symptom of too much estrogen is swelling and tenderness in the breasts. Women experiencing this might also feel bloated, have poor libido, develop fibrocystic lumps in the breasts, and experience hair loss. Headaches and irregular menstrual periods are also common.

On an emotional level, it can cause mood swings, depression, anxiety, panic attacks, and a lowered sense of self-worth.

Thus, women must try to maintain their estrogen level at a good and healthy level for them. As intermittent fasting can influence this level, we can also use it as a tool to improve your estrogen level.

MORE ON THE GROWTH HORMONE

While estrogen is a hormone that is widely known, the growth hormone and the impact it has on the female body are far less publicized. The human growth hormone or HGH, sometimes simply called the GH or growth hormone, is naturally produced in the pituitary gland. During our development, this hormone impacts our growth but also plays a vital role in the development of sexual differentiation. For women, this would mean that it has a contributing role in menstruation, ovulation, pregnancy, and even lactation.

When women experience an optimal level of this hormone, they feel more energetic, have a high libido, enjoy better sleep, have greater mental clarity and memory, enjoy a better overall mood, and get rid of stubborn fat like cellulite and belly fat much faster.

A lack of this hormone results in brittle bones, lower sex drive, weight gain, aging skin, and poor-quality sleep.

While there are ways to treat lowered levels of HGH, intermittent fasting is a natural way to address this concern. The reason fasting helps people to lose weight but still keep their lean muscle mass and increase their metabolism is that it impacts the HGH.

Several studies have shown that through intermittent fasting, you can combat the drop in HGH as you age. This hormone speeds up tissue repair, helps with the breakdown of fat cells and converting them into energy, and aids in releasing fatty acids (HGH & Intermittent Fasting: Can Fasting Increase HGH? 2021).

These studies confirm that intermittent fasting increases the levels of HGH in the human body, and as a result, those who opt for this way of eating experience higher fat burning rates, as they have lower insulin levels coupled with higher HGH.

The lowered insulin levels are because there are now times when they are not eating, and the body is not in a state of digestion all the time. Thus, there is no need for high insulin levels, and as insulin drops, the body burns fat.

As the body has a higher level of HGH, aging takes place at a slower rate. Cell renewal and healing take place faster, leaving you with a healthy and younger appearance.

Lastly, as the release of fat into energy is taking place, and this is a cleaner source of energy, you will feel more energetic.

THE IMPACT ON DIGESTIVE HORMONES

Hormones regulate the entire human body and all the functions that keep you going. This includes the digestive system. Therefore, we need to look at digestive hormones and the impact that intermittent fasting has on these hormones, too.

Digestive hormones or gastrointestinal hormones (GI hormones) are the collective names for a range of hormones that are all linked to the digestive system. They ensure the comprehensive uptake of nutrients from the food we eat and that it benefits our overall well-being on a cellular level. The body secretes these hormones in the enteroendocrine cells that are found in the pancreas, stomach, and small intestine. These hormones are not restricted to glands and can be found across the entire surface of the digestive tract (RVS Chaitanya Koppala, 2017).

While there are several digestive hormones, the two I want to focus on are leptin and pepsin.

Leptin

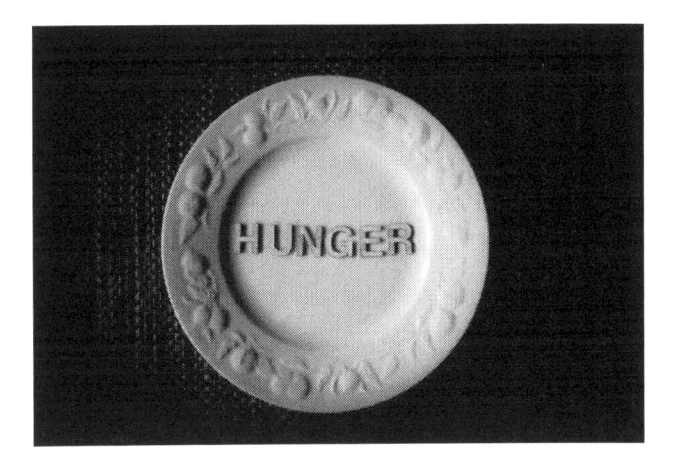

Leptin is the hormone that aids the body in maintaining a balance between the need for food and the amount of energy the body uses. It prevents the body from sending out any messages that you are hungry while you still have plenty of energy resources to provide according to the body's needs. When the leptin levels go too high, the body loses its sensitivity toward leptin and becomes leptin resistant. It means that it can be extremely hard to lose weight as the body will continue to be hungry while it has far more resources than what is necessary. Obesity is not the only medical concern when the body becomes leptin resistant. We also need to look at food addictions, depression, and several neurodegenerative disorders. While fatty liver disease is widely associated with alcoholism, it also presents itself in people who are leptin resistant.

When leptin levels drop below average, it is also not a healthy state to be in. People who have too little leptin easily develop bacterial infections, can also get fatty liver disease, have too much insulin in their bodies, and have lowered sex hormone levels (Leptin: What It Is, Function & Levels, n.d.).

Part of the cause of leptin resistance is increased levels of inflammation in the body. Intermittent fasting can play a helpful role in improving this condition. Once this inflammation is cleared, the body's leptin receptors increase in functionality again and become better at regulating the leptin levels in the body. Not only does this encourage weight loss, but it also reduces the hunger pangs you might constantly feel (Kucine, 2018).

Pepsin

Pepsin is the hormone that is mostly involved in the digestion of protein. For pepsin to work at optimal functionality, it needs an environment that is high in acidity. When the stomach stops receiving food to digest, it alkalizes, and once this happens, the pepsin hormone becomes less active.

Pepsin brings several benefits to the digestive system. It takes a lot of stress off the digestive tract, and it is helpful to treat a leaky gut. It also aids in the secretion of bile and helps to detoxify the liver. However, when pepsin is not functioning as it should, several health concerns can come into play. The one that is widely known as GERD or gastroesophageal reflux disease. This happens when the acid and pepsin levels in the stomach become so high that they leak into the esophagus. GERD is highly uncomfortable to live with, and many other health concerns can ripple from its presence.

Some symptoms of GERD are coughing, a hoarse voice, burning pains in the chest, and the contraction of the vocal cords. This highly acidic secretion can also cause damage to the laryngeal cells.

One way to address this concern is through intermittent fasting, which gives your stomach more downtime and sufficient time to clean itself from any food. Not only can it focus on repairing itself during these times, but it will also lower the production of acid.

Therefore, intermittent fasting is not only one of the most effective long-term solutions to address GERD but also to encourage healing.

INTERMITTENT FASTING–A WAY TO BRING YOUR HORMONES BACK INTO BALANCE

The number of hormonal-caused concerns and how intermittent fasting can aid in treating them is much wider than what I've discussed here. To prevent the book from becoming too complex and using too many medical terms, I've decided to only include the most commonly known challenges. Yet, these should serve as sufficient evidence of how intermittent fasting and giving your body a break from digestion affects so many other hormones that are in control of so many bodily functions, ensuring overall well- being.

4

BUILDING DISCIPLINE

Discipline is the bridge between goals and accomplishment.

— JIM ROHN

KICKSTART CHANGE WITH THE RIGHT MOTIVATION

What is your motivation to start intermittent fasting? Stepping out of our comfort zones is never easy, but it remains necessary to make certain changes if you want to enjoy a different outcome or to change the course of where you are heading. Before we make any changes in life, it is often the case that we need to find ourselves in a position where life is hard, maybe even unbearable. Until that very moment when you realize you are in trouble if you don't change your behavior, it can still be easy to get away with your existing habits.

Thus, I need you to ponder on what is motivating you to make this change. You need to have clarity on what it is that is becoming so hard to deal with that it completely motivates you to jump right in and change your dietary style. For some, it can be an alarming talk with their doctor. Often, we can get away with a certain way of living and eating, but it is when our doctors give us a stern warning or even bad news that we realize that we have to take responsibility for our lives and the future we are creating for ourselves. Numerous health concerns are linked to being overweight, and maybe you are in a desperate state concerning your health. Maybe you want to shed weight to feel more comfortable in your skin and to increase your confidence. Or maybe you just want to feel healthy, enjoy good sleep, and not struggle with any digestive concerns anymore. Whatever your reason is, it might help to write it down; for once matters improve, it's hard to stick to the changes you are making today.

While motivation is a great way to get yourself going, it won't support you in maintaining consistency in the changes you are making. This is mainly because once you feel and look better, the negative side of the situation you were in fades. It is not as uncomfortable anymore, and the worse outcome seems less likely. It is why you need to replace motivation with another driving force that will ensure consistency in what you are doing.

Here, discipline steps in as a major contributing factor toward your success.

HOW TO REMAIN DISCIPLINED IN YOUR INTERMITTENT FASTING

It is easy to state that you need to remain disciplined, but how do you do it, and to what do you stay disciplined? The best way to ensure that you continue to enjoy major benefits from the changes you are making is by incorporating habits into your life. But before I get to this, I want to discuss a few steps you need to take early in the process.

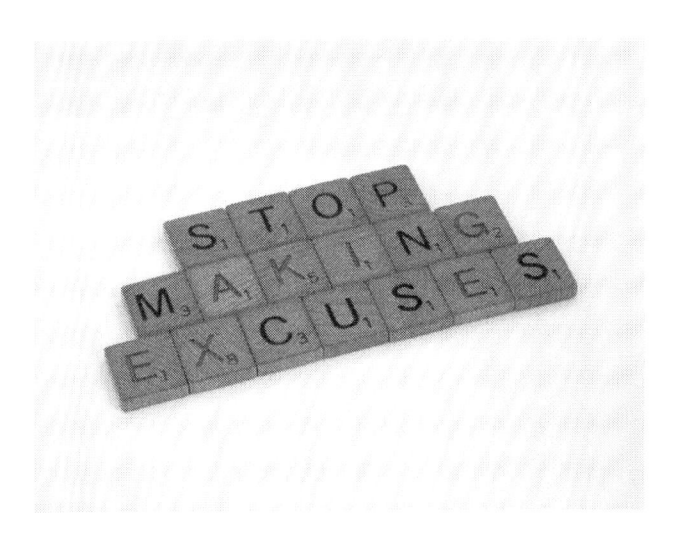

Initially, when we agree to any kind of change, it is exciting. We have hopes and dreams and can see ourselves living a better life. After a while, this vision fades away. It is not enough to keep us going anymore. This is when it becomes important that you've made small habit changes. Thus, let's see how you ensure your dreams of reaping all the benefits that are available when you opt to do intermittent fasting can turn into reality.

Small Habit Changes Can Lead to Outstanding Benefits

I want to recommend that you keep a journal throughout your journey. This book will become your reference that will keep you on track and guide you along the way. There will be days when it is easy to stick to your set eating times, but there will also be days when it is much harder to remain on track, and it is on these days, especially that youwill want to rely on your journal to keep you going.

Know Your Why

This step is an expansion of the first step, determining exactly what motivates you to even consider intermittent fasting as a solution for you. Be clear on what you want to achieve and what the outcome would be if you fail.

Set Your Goals

Whenever we want to achieve greatness in life, it is important to have clarity about what would constitute greatness. Saying you want to lose weight is rather vague. Rather, set a goal weight for yourself. This goal weight should be reasonable; it should be achievable, and it should be something that will truly make a difference in your life.

Another reason it is so important to have a goal in mind is that it will help you know when you've achieved the outcome you desired. Let's say that you want to lose weight and you lose some, but you haven't set a benchmark to measure your success against. You will never experience the feeling that you've achieved your goal. A goal, and especially a goal weight, needs to be measurable. So, as you'll be jotting down a blueprint of your plan and how you will make habit changes in your journal, one of the first things you need to add to your journal is the goal weight that you want to achieve and thus, how much weight you want to lose.

Even if it is not for weight loss that you are opting to give intermittent fasting a fair chance, you still need to be clear on what you want to achieve and how you will know you've achieved it. Say, for example, you want to try intermittent fasting as a means of controlling your blood sugar level. What you are working toward would be a consistent healthy blood sugar level-so; this is what you need to jot down as your goal.

Setting a Time Frame

Humans like to procrastinate. It is mostly when there is no urgency to anything we plan that we simply fail to take the necessary steps. To overcome this, you should set a timeline for yourself. What would be a reasonable time for you to achieve your goal?

Once you have an answer to this question, you need to break this period down into smaller segments. Do this by dividing the total progress you want to make into smaller

milestones. Working from one milestone to the next helps make large goals more achievable. Each minor success not only gives you the confidence to do great things, but also leaves you with a sense of satisfaction and pride for what you've already been able to achieve.

Thus, develop a time frame that is reasonable but not stretched over too long a period. You want to set yourself up for success.

Work Out a Plan

We don't always want to think about what to do, and therefore it is helpful to have a plan in place. Capture your course of action in your journal. How will you start? Maybe at first you will only fast for a few days a week, or if you want to do it daily, maybe opt for a longer time frame to eat in. A good example is to start maybe with a 12-hour window and then plan when you want to increase the span of the fasting times in every 24-hour cycle. If your idea is to get to 16/8 intermittent fasting, how much time needs to pass before you'll be happy to reach this goal? Break this time frame down into smaller bits, and then you'll have a plan about how you should proceed to reach your goal.

Give Yourself Rewards

Sometimes other people acknowledge our successes in life, but if they don't (or even if they do), nothing stops us from celebrating our success ourselves. Thus, reward yourself. If you've reached a set milestone within the period that you've planned to do it in, have a little celebration by rewarding yourself. Maybe buy that book that you want to read or a new piece of clothing that shows off the success you are having. A reward can beanything that makes you feel good.

Remove Triggers and Bad Habits

Habits are nothing but a reaction to a certain trigger. These are often actions that we don't think about at all because we are simply so used to doing certain things when we are confronted with certain triggers. To get rid of behavior that is not supporting your goal and action plan, you need to determine what bad habits you need to replace and what triggers activate this kind of behavior.

First, jot down the bad habits that are holding you back. Maybe you often eat late at night. Maybe you are someone who works long hours and doesn't eat much during the day, but when you are relaxing at night, you like to nibble just before bedtime, ending up sleeping on a full stomach.

When you have identified the bad habits, you need to determine what are the triggers that cause you to behave in that manner. I want to emphasize that these bad habits or mostly actions we perform without thinking because our brains are accustomed to reacting in a certain way when confronted with a certain trigger.

An example would be that you maybe don't want to eat early in the morning, but on your way to work, you walk past a bakery that is surrounded by a cloud of freshly baked goodies, and as you are so used to popping in quickly to grab something that they've just taken hot out of the oven, your stomach is already growling when you are nearing the bakery. The bakery and the aroma of freshly baked goods are the triggers, and your hunger is the response.

Remove the trigger and take a different road to work. This way, you will avoid the trigger that urges you to eat while you are still in your fasting window.

Replace Bad Habits with Good Ones

Many people might say that it is very hard to simply let go of a certain habit. What is easier for many, though, is to replace a bad habit. Let's return to the bakery. Instead of walking into the bakery and buying something freshly baked, you can still walk in and buy a cup of black and unsweetened coffee. This would be perfectly fine to drink while still in your fasting window while you answer the need to go into the bakery to buy something freshly baked. Just make sure that the new habit is not too closely linked to the old habit and that it is not causing unnecessary temptation to give in to your old habit.

TIPS TO HELP YOU STICK TO THIS NEW HABIT

Even when we have a plan in place, it can sometimes be hard to overcome the challenges we set for ourselves. I want you to be successful and reap the positive outcomes you want to enjoy. The following tips will help make it easier to stick to your plans.

Change Your Perspective

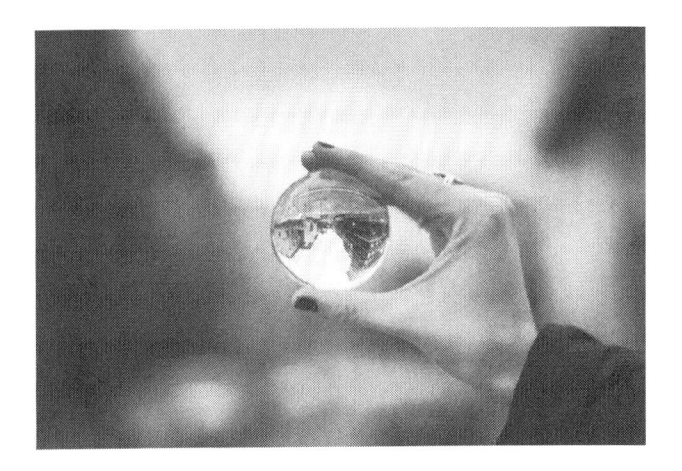

Often, changing your eating habits (especially to lose weight) might feel like a kind of punishment, as if you're denying yourself something that you deserve. This adds such a load of negativity to eating healthy that you are bound to fail at some point. We all feel that there are certain things in life that we deserve, but rather than considering unhealthy food as something you deserve, change your perspective and consider good health and feeling great as something you should have. By making this shift in your perspective, it becomes much easier to stick to your healthy way of eating.

Get a Strategy in Place

The kind of strategy that I am referring to here would be to eat smarter. Certain foods will help you stay feeling full for longer while others just don't. If you normally feel starving when you get up in the morning, but your schedule only allows you to eat a few hours later, the first few hours of your day may be very unpleasant. This is where strategic eating comes in. By making sure that the last meal you eat includes enough whole grains, fiber, and protein, you will feel full for much longer. Drink enough water so that your body remains properly hydrated, and your hunger is bound to be less severe in the mornings. You can also opt to shift your eating window a little. For example, let's say that you are following the 16/8 eating window; if you finish your supper at 7 p.m., you have to wait until 11 a.m. to eat again. If you get up around 6 a.m., it can be five long

hours until you can eat. If you bump your last meal of the day up to 5 p.m., you can break your fast around 9 a.m. This might be a better strategy for you to follow.

Find the Best Solution for You

Intermittent fasting is the kind of solution that works best when you've found the perfect plan to fit into your lifestyle and suit your needs the best. Thus, what I am sharing in this book is an excellent guide to making it work, but you need to continue to experiment with foods and eating schedules that suit your lifestyle and preferences the best to ensure that you reach not only your health goals but also sustain them.

Remain fluid in your ideas regarding eating, and this will help you adapt and adjust your way of eating until you've found the solution that works best for you. Remember that your body, needs, and circumstances can also change over time, and it is best to change your meal times and options to adapt to these changes.

Apply Self-Control

One of the biggest challenges you'll face along your journey is to continue to apply self- control. Self-control can be defined as your ability to control your behavior to achieve your goals, despite having to face temptations. It mostly involves denying yourself instant gratification and resisting urges to do things that would counter your efforts to achieve the desired outcome. Self-control can be a limited resource, and if you don't work on this part of your being to strengthen it, it can run out at some point (Cherry, 2019).

Whether the level of self-control we have is based on our genetics or gained through life experiences is still a topic over which researchers disagree. What they agree on is that there are certain steps you can take to increase the level of self-control you have.

Having better self-control will help you achieve your health objectives, but it will also help you enjoy far greater joy and success in all other aspects of your life (Cherry, 2019).

Change Your Routines

It's easy to fall into certain routines, and, as we are so used to these routines, our brains tell our bodies to respond in a certain manner, as that is what the routine requires from us. If you are in the routine of sitting at night with a cup of tea and a few biscuits while catching up on the day's news before bedtime, you might feel the urge to have a snack late at night, as eating is part of this routine. By changing this routine, you will no longer feel the need to snack late at night because you have removed not only a certain part of the routine but, indeed, your entire routine. This will make it easier to apply self-control and not eat during your fasting window.

Making a Mental Shift

The way you perceive healthy eating will determine in a great way how successful you will be. If you consider healthy eating as a punishment and something that you are forced to do, as the alternative might be some kind of severe or even life-threatening illness, then you might enter the transitioning phase of intermittent fasting with a great deal of resistance toward what you need to do.

Yet, the foundation from where you are starting on this journey can be a much more positively infused one. Rather than seeing it as punishment, consider healthy eating as a form of self-care. You have one body, and the better you look after it, the longer it will last. Just like you have a beauty routine to keep your hair in good health and to keep the wrinkles at bay for as long as you can, eating in a manner that brings about so many health benefits is a way of caring for yourself too. Making this mental shift will help you a lot during this journey, which can be challenging during the early days of intermittent fasting.

Be Kind to Yourself

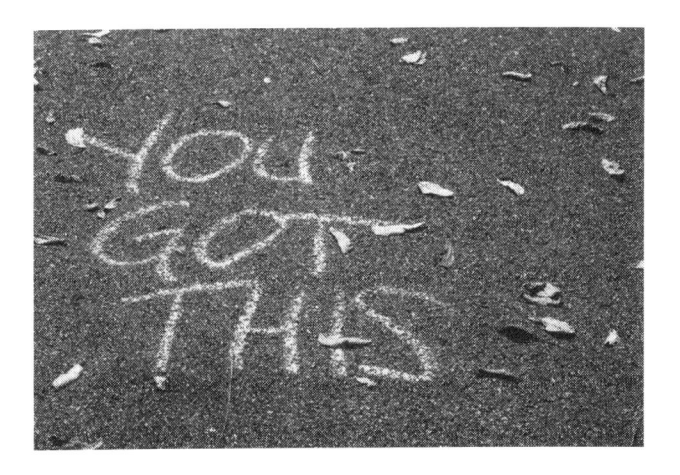

Once you've started this journey, you need to be kind to yourself. There might be days when you fail and do not stick to your eating times. It is during these moments of failure that we can be very harsh on ourselves with criticism. Telling yourself that you are a failure or that you'll never be able to reach your goal will not help you in any way. Rather, choose to be kind to yourself. Treat yourself like you are your own best friend, and while you know that you've failed on this one occasion, consider this only as a lesson learned and let it serve as inspiration to do better next time around.

Take It One Day at a Time

When the journey is hard, focus only on your next step. Don't spend too much time pondering what the outcome could be, how you will persevere, or what you've done over recent days that will prevent you from reaching the goal you desire. Simply take one day at a time. Only focus on getting through one day, and gradually the days will all become easier until the day comes when you can't even imagine yourself eating in any different manner.

Focus on What You Can Eat

The more we focus on the things we can't have, the more we want to have them. The more you focus on the times when you are fasting, the more you will want to eat during

these times. Rather than having thoughts about food consume your mind during your fasting time, spend your time thinking about what you can eat and when you can eat, andhow you will feel when you've completed another day with great success.

Apply Self-Control

One of the biggest challenges you'll face along your journey is to continue to apply self- control. Self-control can be defined as your ability to control your behavior to achieve your goals despite having to face temptations. It mostly involves denying yourself instant gratification and resisting urges to do things that would counter your efforts to achieve the desired outcome. Self-control can be a limited resource, and if you don't work on this part of your being to strengthen it, it can run out at some point (Cherry, 2019).

Whether the level of self-control we have is based on our genetics or through life experiences is still a topic over which researchers disagree. What they do agree on is that there are certain steps you can take to increase the level of self-control you have.

Having better self-control will help you to achieve your health objectives, but it will also help you to enjoy far greater joy and success in all other aspects of your life (Cherry, 2019).

Tips to Increase Your Self-Control

Change Your Attitude

When we go through life seeing ourselves as victims of our circumstances, we employ very little self-control, but when you change your perspective on life and see that you are free to make certain choices and that you are in control of your life, you are bound to be more controlled in your behavior. It boils down to making the shift from seeing yourself as a mere puppet of others and the situation you find yourself in into being the one who calls the shots in your life.

Set Goals

Setting goals, not only regarding your weight but in all other areas in life, will help you to be in greater control, and the more control you feel you have, the more control you will want to gain.

Monitor the Outcome

Take stock of the outcomes you are enjoying. When you are taking deliberate steps to increase the level of self-control you have, you need to monitor the results that you are obtaining. This will guide you to areas where you can still improve and help you to see what you need to do more to bring the kind of outcomes you desire.

Increase Your Confidence

Sometimes we might set out to do something, but deep inside, we are not convinced that we are capable of achieving it. This will weaken our self-control when we are facing temptation. This is when you can reap a lot of benefits from having milestones in place that will lead you toward your goal. Every milestone that you achieve will serve to increase your confidence in the fact that you can achieve your goals, and it will help you to portray far more self-control when you are facing temptation that can easily take you off the track toward success.

Try to Avoid Temptation

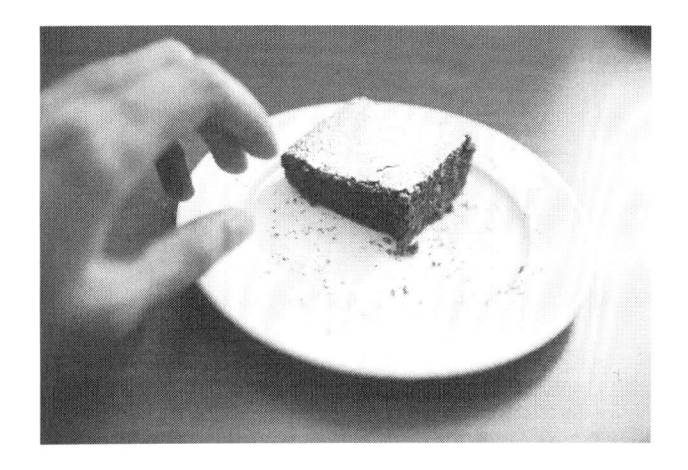

Does the saying, "Don't lead me into temptation for I already know a shortcut," apply to you? If this is the case, then try to avoid temptation as much as possible until you've been able to grow your confidence. If you know that you are going to be tempted to eat during times when you are fasting or attending a certain event, try to avoid going. If you're used to snacking at night, avoid this temptation by cleaning your house with all your favorite snacks. Especially when you are still busy forming your new habits, it is best to avoid any kind of temptation.

Don't Dilute Your Willpower

Self-control feeds off willpower, but willpower is a limited resource that can run out too quickly if we spread it over too many goals at once. It's better to focus on one goal at a time rather than having several things that you want to achieve at once and then not

have the necessary resources to achieve your goals. What can easily happen during these moments is that the first goal fails, and the rest follow like dominos. If your main focus is to get used to intermittent fasting to achieve the outcome you desire, then make this the only goal that you focus on at the time to preserve your willpower for the times when it is necessary.

INTERMITTENT FASTING AND YOUR BUDGET

It is often the case that diets and the food allowed in a certain diet are expensive. This is not the case when it comes to intermittent fasting. The first saving comes in as you will be eating fewer meals a day. A large part of any family's monthly grocery expenses is allocated to snacks. As you will have less time to snack in, you will already be cutting back on this expense.

When you are opting to eat healthily, it doesn't have to be expensive either. Many healthy food sources are far more affordable than processed foods. Stick to raw and whole foods, and you will see how your food budget shrinks, meaning more savings to apply elsewhere. This kind of saving is just one more benefit you can reap from opting to make intermittent fasting a lifestyle you follow.

5

INTERMITTENT FASTING FOR WOMEN BELOW 30

Nature gives you the face you have at twenty; it is up to you to merit the face you have at fifty.

— COCO CHANEL

As a young woman, it is the easiest thing to take your beauty for granted. That youthful and radiant appearance simply comes naturally to you. It is only much later in life that we all, not only women, realize that we should've taken the necessary steps to preserve this beauty for as long as possible. While skincare routines, beauty treatments, and the quality of the beauty products you use play an important role, it is also what we put into our bodies that play a major role in how successful we will be in maintaining this outer appeal. If you want to take the necessary steps to preserve your beauty from a young age onwards, then intermittent fasting is a fantastic way to help achieve this goal.

FINDING THE BEST FASTING SCHEDULE

In chapter 1, I mentioned the 16/8 intermittent fasting method and the 5/2 approach, OMAD, and more extended periods of fasting. I would like to dig a little deeper into what the pros and cons are of these types and explore any other available options. This will provide you with a solid foundation of choices to determine which type of fasting is the best for you and where to start on this journey.

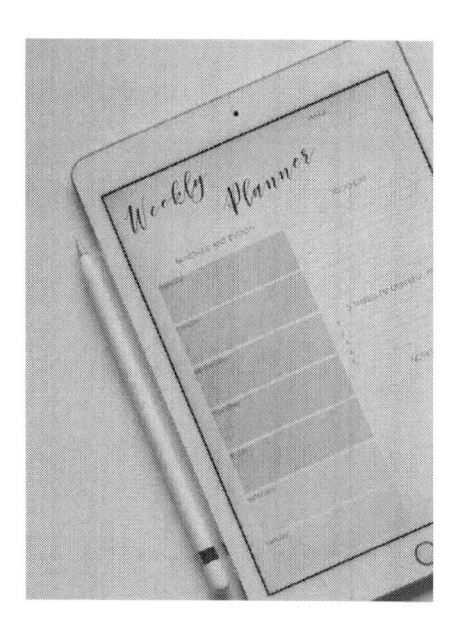

Pros and Cons of 16/8 Intermittent Fasting Period for Your Age Group

I have already said a lot about this type of fasting, so I don't want to expand on this much besides noting that it has several variances. Some prefer to start on this type of fasting as a 12/12 or a 14/10 window. You can even shorten the period you eat more and increase your fasting period to 18/6. It all depends on you and your lifestyle. Many prefer this option, as there are no days that you'll have to go without food or even have to count the calories of your meals. However, this becomes a challenge when you are often out late at night and are used to eating late. Eating a late supper will mean that it can be quite late into the next day before you can eat anything. If you are used to having an early supper and seldom face situations where you will eat late, this shouldn't be a problem for you at all.

Instead of having three meals per day, people following this method usually only eat two meals, and you can still snack if you want to within your eating window.

Pros and Cons of the 5/2 Method for Your Age Group

This can be trickier, for it means that during a week, there would be two 24-hour cycles during which you won't be able to eat at all. Being able to eat only very little for a day can be daunting for many newbies to fasting. Yet, some consider this a minor sacrifice for being able to eat anything they want all the other days of the week. You have the freedom to choose which days you fast and, on your fasting days, the maximum number

of calories allowed is 500 for women. It is why some refer to this eating plan as the modified-calorie intermittent fasting routine.

If this is the method that you find most appealing, it is important to take note that you never have to fast two days in a row, but researchers believe that if you do, the positive effect that it will have on your health is much greater because your body will be a stage of recovery and repair for much longer.

Pros and Cons of OMAD Fasting for Your Age Group

One meal a day fasting is easy to understand. It means that you'll be able to eat only once a day. While highly effective, this is a rather extreme way of fasting and not something I would recommend if you are just starting on this journey. When you have this one meal that is allowed in 24 hours, there are no restrictions on what you may eat.

If this is the solution you choose, you must consume enough fluids to ensure that your body remains hydrated. You can drink as much water and unsweetened and milk-free tea and coffee as you like.

A ripple effect of this way of eating is that consuming all the calories your body needs per day during one meal is very hard. Thus, people who follow this routine consume far fewer calories daily, and it results in substantial weight loss. As a result, some may experience a drop in their blood sugar levels, which represents itself as a drop in their energy levels.

While you can consume this one meal any time during the day, it is best not to eat it straight before bedtime. As your only meal per day, it is more than likely very calorie-rich, and you need to give your body time to digest the food before entering the resting phase. While effective, it is not a sustainable solution over extended periods.

Pros and Cons of Alternate Day Fasting for Your Age Group

This fasting method is in many ways similar to the 5/2 method. The difference is that during the 5/2 method, you'll be consuming only 500 calories two days per week, while following this method will only consume 500 calories every second day. It means that one day you will eat normally, and the next, you will consume far fewer calories and then return to a day of normal eating again and repeat. This way, you give

your body has plenty of time to recover and restore itself by having enough resources to takecare of cell renewal that slows down aging.

The secret to success with this plan is to remain consistent. It can be a sustainable solution that will deliver many health benefits if you do.

CHOOSING THE BEST FASTING FOUNDATION

When you are still younger than 30 and trying intermittent fasting for the first time, it is important to create a sustainable foundation for yourself. Take your time and try a few methods to see which option works the best for you, and once you have one that is suitable for your lifestyle and is sustainable for you, you know that you have a platform to work from for the rest of your life.

INTERMITTENT FASTING AND EXERCISE

The biggest concern that many women have when they are considering fasting is whether they can exercise while they are not eating. The good news is, yes, you can. Exercise will benefit your body in many ways, and I will never recommend that you stop doing it.

Here too, you need to find the workout that suits your body the best.

If you are already following an exercise regime, then there is no reason you can't continue with it. It might just be a case of shifting your exercise schedule around a bit to ensure that none of the negative effects that some people experience while exercising during fasting becomes a concern to you. One of these would be to exercise after you've eaten rather than at the end of your fasting window. Say you are used to exercising first thing in the morning. Being at the end of your fasting window, you might feel light-headed or low on energy. Rather, settle for a time when you have eaten and have enough energy to do so.

If you ever feel bad during your exercise routine, stop immediately and give your body the time it needs to recover.

Take care that you have enough fluids while exercising. You will lose a lot of fluid during your exercise regime and must replenish these fluids.

Strength Training and HIIT

During strength training, you are building your muscle mass. This is an amazing way to combat any chance of experiencing loss of muscle during fasting. It is best to schedule such a workout session right before your fasting window ends and then eat immediately after your training or train during your eating window. Make sure you eat proteins and complex carbs before or after your training.

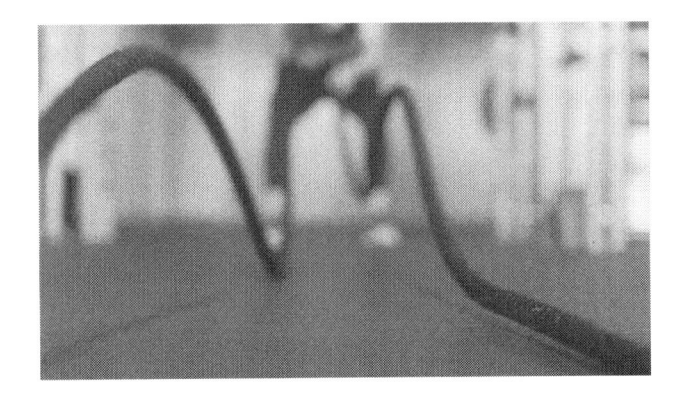

Remain aware of what your body is telling you throughout your entire workout session, and you will be able to do any level of strenuous workout.

Exercising for Low Energy Levels

While you should never push your body beyond what it is capable of, you must do some kind of exercise. Thus, if you are just starting an exercise routine or are feeling low on energy, you can opt for various forms of low-intensity workouts like yoga or barre. If you don't feel all that great during your first weeks of fasting, taking part in a barre class regularly might even help you feel better much sooner.

Lastly, never underestimate walking as a highly effective and powerful exercising method. Walking has minimal impact on the body, and while it increases your heart rate, it never puts your body under any stress.

TIPS TO HELP MAKE YOUR EXERCISE REGIME EASY

Suppose you are completely new to intermittent fasting and are trying this as a weight and health management solution for the first time, and you would like to include regular exercise as part of your health action plan. In that case, I have a few tips to make it all easier.

Start Slowly

Our bodies adjust quickly to what we expose them to, especially while we are still young, but don't overdo it. Starting slowly gives your body enough time to get used to all the changes, and this will become a sustainable habit.

Find the Best Time of Day

Suppose you are used to doing HIIT training early in the morning and when fasting, this will fall into your fasting window. In that case, you will most likely struggle to get through your regime. So, change your exercising time or fasting window. Suppose there is no other time for you to exercise than during this period. In that case, it might be beneficial to shift your fasting period so that you can eat right before or after you've exercised.

Enjoy Variety

There are several types of exercise that you can do. Exercise doesn't have to be high intensity. Start with something simple and easy that you can keep up with easily, rather than jumping all in at a level that is too demanding and forces you to give up early. Mixing things up is an easy way to enjoy the benefits of all kinds of exercise. Some days you can do high-intensity workouts and stick to something far easier.

Replenish Your Electrolytes

A solution that will help you make exercising easier during your fasting windows is to hydrate with fluids that are high in electrolytes and low in calories. Some good choices are natural sports drinks or even coconut water.

As long as you are responsible for your exercise regime, it is perfectly fine to continue to exercise, stay fit, increase your endorphins, and enjoy overall health and well-being.

FASTING TO MANAGE YOUR WEIGHT

As women age, the harder it becomes to shed their extra weight. This is quite simply how the biology of the human body works. Therefore, when women are in their twenties, they are in a time that is still considered a period when it is relatively easy to lose weight. Still, intermittent fasting is widely considered the most effective method if your goal is to lose weight through this new way of eating.

This method is the 16/8 method. There are several reasons this is such a popular method of intermittent fasting. The first reason is that it is very sustainable. Many diets are highly effective and bring about a lot of weight loss, but as they are too demanding or extreme, they aren't sustainable. This often results in picking up all the weight again and, in some cases, becoming heavier than before.

The 16/8 method is easy to ease into. You should never consider the 16/8 fasting method as a diet, but rather a lifestyle. Combining it with any exercise regime or diet is easy to speed up your weight loss and enjoy even greater results.

The method is flexible, and you have a choice over when you want to eat and when you want to fast. While the most common routine would be to have an early supper and then only eat again later in the morning the next day, you can opt to eat early and have your last meal during the late afternoon. This flexibility is even easier to enjoy if you are single or do not have to care for your family.

As this method doesn't require any calorie counting, you can indulge at times in unhealthy foods without guilt. While the results you will enjoy from eating healthy during the eating window are far better if you don't, it won't break your entire routine.

This style of restricted eating has many attributes that are closely linked to the keto diet, and you can reap many of the same benefits as you could enjoy when opting for keto. The difference is when you are following the keto diet, you are forcing your body into a state of ketosis by consuming a very low percentage of carbohydrates while eating more foods high in fats. Ketosis means your body is burning fat cells for fuel rather than operating on glucose. Intermittent fasting also forces your body into ketosis as a result of the lack of glucose in the bloodstream. When your body burns fat, you will enjoy a much more stable flow of energy and not endure any slumps or feel sleepy.

This process is called metabolic switching, and while this is a good thing when you want to enjoy weight loss, it is something you need to monitor if you are suffering from type 1 diabetes, a topic we'll discuss next.

FASTING FOR DIABETES

Intermittent fasting and diabetes are two very intertwined topics. By restricting the times you eat, you directly affect your hormones, and the hormones linked to diabetes are most likely the ones that are the most affected. As this effect is so great, the question often arises whether intermittent fasting is even safe for those who are diagnosed with diabetes.

While this concern is related mostly to type 1 diabetes, it is safe to opt for intermittent fasting to address the concerns linked to both types of diabetes as long as you do it in collaboration with your medical professional as part of a comprehensive and balanced plan.

As it is far more common that people develop type 2 diabetes at a more mature age, I want to focus in this section mostly on the impact that intermittent fasting has on type 1 diabetes, as this is commonly diagnosed during the teen and preteen years.

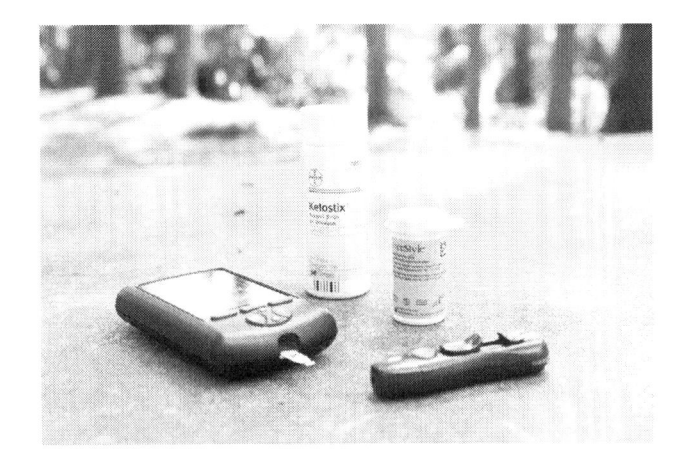

Until recently, the focus of the medical research world was mostly on the impact, benefits, and risks that go along with using intermittent fasting as a way to address concerns when it comes to type 2 diabetes. Now, the focus has shifted, and more research studies are trying to explore how intermittent fasting can be beneficial to people suffering from type 1 diabetes.

While there have mostly only been animal studies to date, it appears that through the weight loss achieved through intermittent fasting, type 1 diabetes patients enjoy an improvement in their condition. This way of eating also increases the insulin sensitivity of these patients, which is also helpful in diabetes management. Another benefit that became evident is that intermittent fasting has a positive impact on the renewal of damaged pancreas cells. While more studies would be necessary to determine conclusive results, the outcome appears to be promising (WeCareBlog, 2021).

While we have these potential benefits, on the one hand, the other holds onto several risks involved for these patients if they take on intermittent fasting without necessary caution.

Many of the medications often prescribed to patients with type 1 diabetes promote water loss in the body. So, patients are more prone to suffering from dehydration, and by eating only during a certain interval of the day, the risk of dehydration is much higher for these patients. It is why it is so important that these patients ensure to consume enough fluids even during their fasting phase.

Treatment for type 1 diabetes patients is very specific to the individual. The dosages of their medications are closely linked to their dietary habits. If patients change their way of eating as dramatically as implementing intermittent fasting without also changing their dosages under the guidance of their doctor, it can lead to hypoglycemia. This happens because treatment is still ensuring sufficient insulin in the cells to address the

level of glucose present, but because of fasting, this level of glucose is no longer present in the cells.

Lastly, the risk for ketoacidosis increases as the body is now breaking down fat cells because of the lack of glucose in the bloodstream or when the prescribed dosage of insulin is still linked to a former way of eating and is now too high (WeCareBlog, 2021).

When we look at what expert organizations in the field have to say about intermittent fasting and type 1 diabetes, it becomes clear that they don't advise against it or in its favor. This poses the question of how you can opt for intermittent fasting when you are a diabetes type 1 patient.

TIPS FOR SAFE INTERMITTENT FASTING FOR TYPE 1 DIABETES PATIENTS

- Always change your way of eating under the supervision of your medical professional.
- Monitor your blood sugar level regularly, ensuring that it never drops too low.
- Familiarize yourself with the symptoms of hypoglycemia so that you can take the necessary steps in time to prevent it from happening.
- If you have a prescribed insulin pump, make sure to address changes in the dosages and intervals that you need to use your pump with your physician.
- Don't be too stuck to your eating window. If your blood sugar level drops too low while fasting, you must break your fast and eat something.
- Start slowly. Making any radical changes can cause more harm than good.

If you are a type 2 diabetes patient, please explore the section focusing on type 2 diabetes and intermittent fasting in the next chapter.

INTERMITTENT FASTING AND LASTING YOUTH AND BEAUTY

It is often the case with humankind that we only value the things only we had once we've lost them. This can be true for loved ones, friendships, good health, and also our youthful appearance. However, when it comes to lasting youth and beauty, there is an

awakening taking place in the younger generation of women across the globe to start early on, taking the necessary steps to preserve their beauty for as long as possible.

While you are still in your twenties, you are most likely going through a phase where you are strengthening the foundation on which you are building your life. This foundation has demanded in the fields of work and your career, as well as love and finding a partner with whom you want to grow old. It is a time when the level of confidence you have will be a determining factor in how successful you'll be in achieving your goals.

One of the most effective ways to increase your confidence is to ensure that you are looking good. Everyone is blessed with a certain kind of beauty, and it is up to you how long you can preserve this beauty and how confident you are in your appearance.

It is not only how good you look that contributes to your level of confidence, though, but also the degree to which you apply self-care. Through self-care, you can be sure that you are taking the necessary steps to preserve your physical, mental, and emotional health and that you will remain radiant for much longer. While there are plenty of beauty products on the market that will assist you in this quest, it is often self-care through maintaining a balance in your life, spending time with yourself, regular exercise, eating healthy, and getting enough quality sleep that delivers the greatest contribution.

Intermittent fasting plays an important role as it assists with preserving the beauty and a youthful appearance as well as maintaining overall health and well-being. While it is a way to manage your weight, intermittent fasting also helps to speed up the metabolism, which increases the rate at which cell renewal takes place. Fasting also triggers autophagy (Schneider, 2020).

All You Need to Know About Autophagy

While widely unknown, the term autophagy plays an important role in aging. Every moment of our lives, we have cells that are damaged or old and then die. Autophagy is the scientific name for the body's ability to clear itself of dead cells and damaged protein. The clearing process is necessary as it is the only way there will be room for new cells to develop. It is a completely natural process, and it is just how the body operates, but you have a certain level of control over how effective the process is. Researchers determined a link between the rate at which autophagy takes place and weight management, insulin control, and a reduction in the prevalence of certain cancers and even heart disease.

These diseases occur when your body is not getting rid of dead cells at the same rate it used to when you are younger, and the dead cells start to clog up certain renewal

processes. It prevents cell division as it should take place, and this results in aging, but also age-related diseases, and cells can even become cancerous (Schneider, 2020).

In short, autophagy plays a major role in how long you will look and feel young and healthy, when certain ailments will present themselves, and ultimately how long you will live. By having the process function at an optimal rate, you can enjoy better brain health for much longer, sustain a healthy weight, experience less inflammation in your body, and age in a healthy manner (Schneider, 2020).

What is the link between intermittent fasting and increasing the level of autophagy in your body?

"Intermittent fasting is a possible way to induce autophagy. Under normal conditions, when the cell has sufficient nutrients, autophagy degrades damaged components in the cell. When fasting starves the cells, autophagy helps digest some of the cell components, to provide the necessary energy for survival" (Davis, 2021 para 11).

Autophagy and ketosis (when your body breaks down fat cells into ketones as its primary energy source) are closely linked. Intermittent fasting can slow down the pace at which your body ages, allowing you to enjoy a youthful appearance and lasting health. While you can reap many benefits from the process and the speedy cell renewal on the inside, you also notice that process taking place on the outside, as you'll be able to enjoy radiant and healthy skin for much longer.

As we age, our skins become less elastic and produce less oil, resulting in dry skin often presenting itself as wrinkles. Coupled with the slower production of collagen and a slowed pace of getting rid of dead skin cells, the appearance of wrinkles worsens. It is why using intermittent fasting to get rid of your dead skin cells will help to maintain a radiant appeal, too.

Intermittent fasting, or any other step that you take to preserve your youthful appearance for longer during your twenties, will most likely only show reward during the years to come. While it might feel unnecessary at a younger age to take all these steps, it will be something you will be grateful for in the years to come as you mature.

As a woman in your twenties, there is indeed a range of benefits you can enjoy from intermittent fasting that will affect a wide range of areas in your life.

6

INTERMITTENT FASTING FOR WOMEN IN THEIR 30S AND 40S

You can't really be present for the people in your life if you aren't taking care of yourself.

— KERRY WASHINGTON

In this chapter, I want to touch on several biological changes that occur in women when they move into their 30s and 40s. Throughout, it is important to remember that there is no set time when these changes occur, and for some women, some changes happen earlier than others. Maybe you are experiencing some of these changes only in your 50s. What I am providing, though, is a general idea of the maturing process for women to provide a platform from which to explore the impact of intermittent fasting.

THE MOST PREDOMINANT CHANGES IN WOMEN 30 YEARS AND OLDER

Some changes I expand on will be visible, some not, some might become a matter of immediate concern, while others might already be developing only to rear ahead much later on in life.

Weight Gain

While weight management might be a problem for some women throughout their entire lives, others only struggle to get rid of excess weight later on in life, especially after turning 30. At this age, weight continues to increase on the hips and thighs for most women. While this increase in size can negatively affect your health and the level of joy you experience in life, it is mostly the kind of weight gain that presents itself at a much later stage in life that is a matter of great concern. I am referring to weight gain around the belly area. Belly fat or visceral fat is a form of high-risk fat, bringing along a range of health concerns.

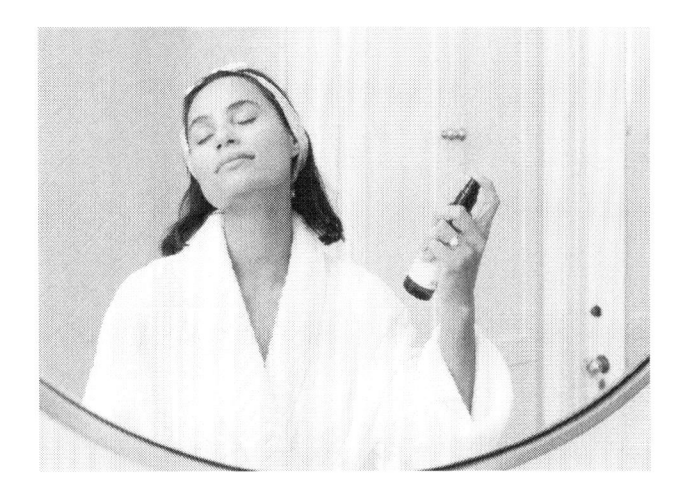

Changes in Skin

While crows' feet and laugh lines will present themselves already during this stage in a woman's life, the skin maintains its thickness until about 50. From then onward, the skin gets thinner and far less elastic. While this might appear to be a challenge to confront only, later on, the results you will have at a later stage largely depend on how you take care of your skin during your 30s and 40s.

Bone Density

Some of the internal changes taking place in a woman's body are the reduction in bone density. Bone density continues to increase until about the age of 30. After about the age of 35, bones become less dense, increasing the risk of osteoporosis and sustaining bone fractures. While the process starts already in the 30s, it speeds up after menopause. It is why it is such an important time to take care of bone density by living a healthy lifestyle, getting enough exercise, and doing some strength training.

Heart Health

Estrogen plays a vital role in sustaining heart health as it keeps the artery walls flexible (Canyon Ranch, n.d.). Heart disease is much more common in women than what is widely assumed. While this is another concern that plays a much bigger role only after menopause, now is the time to take action to reduce your chances of experiencing this kind of medical concern.

THE BENEFITS OF INTERMITTENT FASTING DURING THE 30S AND 40S

It is still not too late to make a difference to your health and overall well-being if you fall into this age range and haven't been taking care of your health until now. I want to urge you that if this is you, do not wait any longer to take steps to reverse the effect of aging, and do not wait until you are confronted with one of the medical concerns already mentioned before you take any action.

16/8 Fasting in Your 30s and 40s

This is still the easiest way to start with intermittent fasting, and if you are completely new to the concept of fasting, then it is the best place to start. As previously suggested, start by easing into the routine and give the habit of eating only at certain times the opportunity to set in. You can also start by opting for a 12/12 schedule and gradually work your way toward 16/8 or even 18/6, as long as you take steps that are sustainable for your lifestyle.

The benefits that you'll reap are that it is relatively easy to sustain this way of eating and, without denying yourself any food, you will lose weight as you'll be consuming fewer calories. Even for women who have families, this remains the most practical solution to shed extra weight and, even better, keep it off.

While this way of fasting will bring about weight loss and far better weight management in the long-term, you will also enjoy the benefits of slowed aging, increased metabolism

during a time when your metabolism is slowing down and more effective cell renewal, preventing premature aging.

5/2 Fasting in Your 30s and 40s

This method is also relatively easy to sustain, especially if it is your responsibility to take care of the diet of others too, like when cooking for a family. It is not as restrictive, and you can eat anything you like except on the days when you are limiting your calories. You also have the choice of deciding which two days will fit the best into your schedule.

Alternate Day Fasting in Your 30s and 40s

This is another sustainable way to take control of your weight and overall health and well-being. As it is relatively easy to follow and is based on the same principles as the 5/2 fasting method, you will reap the same kind of benefits. Remember that the only difference between the 5/2 method and the alternate-day fasting method is that with the latter, you will restrict the calories you'll be consuming every second day.

Juicing Fast in Your 30s and 40s

Until now, I haven't yet mentioned juice fasting. Juice fasting refers to a certain period, often ten days, during which you only drink freshly pressed juice. This will be the juice of fruits and vegetables with no additives or even fiber from the fruit or vegetable. It results in a far lower calorie intake, and while it is not sustainable, you can opt to incorporate this more drastic type of dieting in combination with any of the more sustainable solutions previously mentioned.

Juice fasting is something I would only recommend when you are already in the habit of following one of the other methods of intermittent fasting.

The benefits of this kind of fasting are far more than mere extreme weight loss. Freshly pressed juice contains all the vitamins and minerals that your body needs, but it requires very little digestion, as you will only consume liquids. This type of fasting increases your energy levels and, as juice is high in antioxidants, it cleanses your body from toxins and

clears up inflammation in the body. Juice fasts also strengthen the immune system as it is so loaded with vitamins.

While you are on this type of fasting, your gut health will improve as it brings back the balance of good and bad bacteria in the gut. Over recent years, researchers have been focusing on the vital role that the gut plays in our overall well-being, including our mental health. Going through this kind of fasting will most likely also improve your emotional state.

The cons linked to this kind of fasting are that it is quite severe and that you will most likely gain the weight that you've lost once you eat again. Therefore, it is so important that you only opt for this drastic measure when you are already managing your weight with one of the more sustainable fasting methods.

Water Fasting

This is another drastic version of fasting and should never last over 72 hours. During this time, you will not be having any teas or coffees and no food at all. You are only allowed to drink water and lots of it. As your body won't be involved in any kind of digestion during this period, it provides an optimal opportunity to cleanse the system and invigorate cell renewal. While you can do this regularly, you must do this as part of another fasting method.

During this period, it is so important to ensure that you hydrate enough and drink between two and three liters of water per day to help your body get rid of all the toxins it will release during this time.

While water fasting brings about an increase in weight loss, it is not sustainable, and you need to return to a less severe weight management plan afterward.

Some people prefer to kick off a weight management plan with water fast, while others prefer to first get accustomed to eating only during certain intervals rather than jumping into the deep end first. The choice remains yours, as you know how well you do with eating restrictions. Water fasting can be beneficial, but please do so with caution.

FASTING TIPS IN YOUR 30S AND 40S

When you've reached this age group, you've likely already started to experience fluctuations in your hormonal levels, even more so if you haven't been part of any other weight management plan during your 20s.

Be Aware of Hormonal Changes

That's why it is important that when you decide to do intermittent fasting for the first time, you need to do so with a great awareness of any changes you might experience. Any major changes to your diet can, and most likely will, affect your hormones, and if you notice any changes that make you feel uncomfortable, you need to discuss this with your doctor.

Eat Enough Protein

Losing muscle mass is part of aging, and if you are going to lower your intake of proteins, the odds are that you might speed up the undesired process. It is why you need to take care to consume enough protein-rich foods during your eating window. Including sufficient protein sources in your diet coupled with exercise will combat the effect of muscle loss.

Always Hydrate

I've mentioned that when skin ages, it loses its elasticity and ability to hold enough moisture. It is why you need to ensure that you flush your body with enough water to stay hydrated. Dry skin is more prone to wrinkles and premature aging.

EXERCISE AND INTERMITTENT FASTING IN YOUR 30S AND 40S

If you've been active all your life, then this is not a topic of any genuine concern to you. Then, my only advice would be to continue doing what you are doing, for exercise brings about far greater benefits than merely being fit once you reach this age. Bone density is one of the several benefits you'll enjoy if you are staying fit through regular exercise.

If you haven't been doing any or very little exercise until now, my suggestion is to start slowly, especially if you are already busy fasting.

Choose forms of exercise that are low impact, like walking, yoga, or barre. As you get fitter and your body is more used to it, you can include more strenuous forms of exercise.

THE BEST WAY TO LOSE WEIGHT FAST

Losing weight can be more challenging in this particular age group, but as this will only get harder in the future, it is best to start right away. The most sustainable methods in intermittent fasting will always be 16/8, 5/2, or alternate-day fasting. It is why I will always recommend that you follow any of these three methods for sustained weight loss and to better manage your weight over time.

However, maybe you are not experiencing the degree of weight loss that you've been hoping for, or you need to lose more weight quickly and keep it off afterward. In this case, I would recommend that you opt for a juice or even water fast, or even alternate between the two types of fasting, as they both bring about different benefits.

When you are done with either of these options, return to one of the sustainable solutions and not regular eating. While these more drastic forms of fasting will cause weight loss of a greater significance, the other three more sustainable methods will ensure that you continue to shed the extra weight, or at least that you don't gain back any of the weight that you've lost during the shorter and more impactful forms of fasting.

It will also help to include at least one form of exercise while you are fasting. This will bring about a different number of benefits that will not only improve your physical well- being but also contribute to your mental and emotional wellness.

Another way to ensure weight loss that will deliver lasting results is by resetting your metabolism. I often hear women complain they are gaining weight in their 30s and 40s while their eating habits haven't changed at all since their 20s. While their eating habits might not have changed, their bodies surely are showing signs indicating it is aging.

One unpleasant thing about aging is that the metabolic rate slows down. To better understand how to combat this, we need to be clear on what the metabolic rate is.

Metabolism refers to the chemical processes that take place inside our bodies and what is quite simply keeping us alive and well. The fuel for this process is calories, and the faster this metabolic rate is, the more calories you will burn just to sustain your body every day. When metabolism starts to slow down, it requires fewer calories, and while you are eating as you've always done, your body is now storing the excess calories as fat. Hence, you are picking up weight even though you haven't changed your eating habits.

Four Factors Determining Metabolic Rate

Normal Activity Level

The first is your activity level through daily activities or exercise. If you spend most of your day sitting behind a computer, you are bound to burn fewer calories than when you are in an active position and mostly spend time on your feet. If you do regular exercise, you will also burn calories at a higher rate. Thus, the more active you are, the more calories you'll burn and the higher your metabolism will be.

The Thermic Effect of Food

The thermic effect of food, or TEF, refers to how many calories your body burns during the digestive process. Some foods (mostly processed foods) contain a high number of calories and require very little digestion, while other foods require a lot of digestion and are low in calories. We sometimes refer to these foods as negative-calorie foods. Whether they are truly negative-calorie is a matter for debate, but what I want to get across is that there are foods that require a lot of calories for digestion and are low in the number of calories they contain, and these foods are mostly raw vegetables that are high in fiber.

Resting Metabolic Rate

Resting metabolic rate, or RMR is another factor in your metabolism. We forget that our bodies burn calories even while we are sleeping. During our resting phase, the body is very busy with processes like cell regeneration and repair. It is also when it cleanses the system from toxins, and it requires calories to fulfill these tasks. The rate at which your body burns calories during this phase is the RMR.

Non-Exercise Activity Thermogenesis

Lastly, NEAT stands for non-exercise activity thermogenesis. It is the rate at which we burn calories that are not used for exercise but merely by being awake; say, for example, how many calories you burn while sitting on the sofa watching your favorite series.

When these rates at which your body burns calories slow down, it is indicative that your overall metabolism is slowing down due to age, loss in muscle mass, changes in your hormones, and factors like stress, pollution, and poor-quality sleep.

While increasing your muscle mass through resistance training, increasing the demand for calories through more exercise, and eating the foods that require a lot of calories for digestion will all help to prevent this slowing-down process from occurring, fasting can also be very beneficial. According to studies, fasting for short periods can increase your metabolism. While fasting for long periods can put your body into starvation mode and slow down your metabolism at an even faster speed, it is now known that temporary boosts of fasting can increase your metabolic rate by as much as 14% (West, 2021).

Thus, while you will lose weight because of consuming fewer calories, you are also encouraging your body to burn calories at a faster rate, combatting the slowing-down process so widely familiar to this age group.

FASTING FOR DIABETES IN YOUR 30S AND 40S

While doctors mostly diagnose type 1 diabetes during the teenage years, the 30s and 40s is the age group when most people start to develop type 2 diabetes. I want to emphasize the fact that not everyone who has type 2 diabetes is overweight, but according to research, as many as 95% of all people in the US who have type 2 diabetes are overweight or live an inactive lifestyle (Dansinger, 2007). When you have type 2 diabetes, your body is still producing insulin but is no longer capable of recognizing it and using this hormone effectively, or it is not producing enough of it.

It is important to understand the role of insulin in the body. The body breaks down all food sources into the smallest kind of energy form: glucose. Glucose is necessary for all bodily functions and is therefore present in your bloodstream. Insulin plays a regulatory role and manages the level of glucose in your bloodstream. If the body is not using glucose optimally or is not producing enough of it, the glucose levels in the bloodstream become too high. A glucose level of 126 milligrams per deciliter of blood or higher after the person has eaten nothing for eight hours will cause a positive diagnosis of type 2 diabetes (Dansinger, 2007).

During intermittent fasting, it is not only the accompanying weight loss that often helps to improve the symptoms or even prevent a positive diagnosis, but it also reduces the glucose levels in the bloodstream, as the body is now forced into a state where it burns fat cells for energy.

The risk involved for type 2 diabetes patients when they are using intermittent fasting as a way to treat their medical concerns is that without adjusting their prescription, the glucose levels can drop to a level that is too low. This is a state of hypoglycemia. It goes along with dizziness, headaches, and feelings of hunger.

While intermittent fasting can be a fantastic way to improve your type 2 diabetes and lose weight, you need to start the process with the support and guidance of your medical professional. This way, you will better monitor your symptoms and see if there is an improvement in your condition, and adjust your prescription according to your new way of eating.

As always, it is best not to make any drastic changes and ease into the process gently. I would suggest that you follow the 16/8 method, but start with maybe only a 12-hour fasting period initially and gradually extend the period during which you will fast.

HOW FASTING CAN IMPROVE YOUR MENTAL AND EMOTIONAL STATE

While many people would frown upon a statement that the 30s and 40s are when the midlife begins, studies dating as far back as 2010 already revealed that many people feel their 30s are the unhappiest decade in their lives. This is often because of unmet expectations, work stress, and pressure to perform, finding a partner, and gain financial security ("Mid-Life Crisis Begins in the Mid-30s, Relate Survey Says," 2010).

The premature mid-life crisis has different origins for men and women. We can narrow the factors that often affect women down to mainly three causes.

Physiological Origins

While menopause starts somewhat later, perimenopause can already start to have an effect. This is due to declining levels of both estrogen and progesterone. Some symptoms

that go along with this reduction in hormones are poor sleeping habits, tiredness, gaining excess weight, anxiety, and experiencing a loss of joy for things they loved before.

Emotional Origins

It can be harder to compete in the workplace and to get to the position you want to be in or maintain your current role. For many women, this is also an age when they want to re-enter the workforce, but as they now have to compete with younger and often very attractive candidates, it can be challenging. This kind of rejection can be emotionally draining and holds the potential to affect a woman's self-esteem negatively.

Societal Origins

It is nothing new that society chases a youthful appearance. Even more mature women are often exposed to models that are their own age. While deep down, it is evident that they are not on the same playing field as the models presented in fashion magazines, often half their age, it can hurt self-esteem. While more mature women bring far more than good looks to the table, it might be daunting to present your experience in a certain field if you are competing with some more attractive candidates.

Intermittent fasting during these years brings some major benefits to your overall health and well-being. Through this type of fasting, you can do more than merely shed weight, which will already boost your state of well-being and your overall self-esteem. It will also increase your energy levels, making you feel more capable of dealing with the challenges that life is presenting you. The fact that it triggers autophagy is worth a mention again, as well as the fact that studies show that after about three months of intermittent fasting, women felt far less depressed, experienced less tension, and could handle emotions such as anger and frustration far better (7 Incredible Things Intermittent Fasting Does for Your Brain, 2020). It is a wonderful way to apply self-care that will hit the brakes on aging and leave the woman in her 30s or 40s feeling far more empowered and ready to deal with any challenge this period in her life might bring about.

7

INTERMITTENT FASTING FOR WOMEN 50 AND OVER

You can't help getting older, but you don't have to get old.

— GEORGE BURNS

For some, turning 50 is a milestone, while others wouldn't dare to make their age known once they reach the big five-zero. How well you've looked after your health and well- being until this point will determine to a great extent how enjoyable you'll find this new period in your life.

If you've been too busy all your life to even consider making healthier choices and your health is only becoming a concern to you now, don't stress. There is still time to make an impact and improve your overall well-being. Taking a holistic approach to your well- being will bear the most positive results. So, start eating healthy, shed that extra weight, get some exercise, and bring balance to your life.

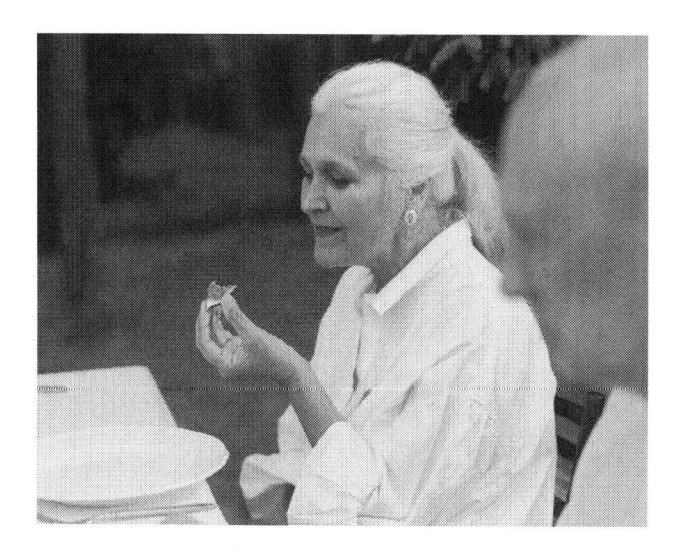

For women in this age category, the most common reasons, after any possible health concerns, for why they are exploring intermittent fasting for the first time would be to lose weight that is now far more challenging to get rid of than ever before and to slow down aging. The good news is that both of these outcomes are achievable through intermittent fasting.

THE BENEFITS OF INTERMITTENT FASTING OVER 50

While we have already discussed the benefits linked to intermittent fasting, I do want to highlight several benefits that are far more applicable to women of a more mature age.

Increasing Brain Power

While getting forgetful is part of getting older, you can control the rate at which this takes place. Studies indicate that when we live off a diet that contains high volumes of sugars and carbs, it increases the speed at which memory loss takes place. Even worse is that it can contribute to dementia. This is often the effect of having persistent high glucose levels. The best way to address this concern is to follow a dietary style where you decrease your glucose levels at some point.

This is not only possible but also effective when you decide to include intermittent fasting in your lifestyle. During your fasting phase, the glucose levels in your bloodstream drop, and your body turns stored fat cells into ketones that serve as the primary energy source during this phase. Ketones are considered a much cleaner form of energy, and, as they produce less reactive oxygen species, the brain benefits from this source of energy (Intermittent Fasting Benefits for Seniors, n.d.).

Improved Circadian Rhythm

Circadian rhythm is a matter of much greater concern to more mature people. It refers to the rhythm dictating all other physical processes that take place in the body which are necessary for survival. The list of processes includes controlling body temperature, sleep schedules, and all other functions vital for survival. The rhythm runs on a 24-hour cycle. If the rhythm is slightly off, it can have a holistic impact, and one way you can reset your circadian rhythm is through intermittent fasting (Intermittent Fasting Benefits for Seniors, n.d.).

Better Heart Health

Increased weight, high blood pressure, high cholesterol levels, and insulin resistance are all health concerns that appear more frequently from the age of 50 years and onwards. Simply by opting for intermittent fasting, you can address these concerns. By allowing for a fasting period in a 24-hour cycle, you can lower your cholesterol and blood pressure, lose unhealthy weight, and improve the body's sensitivity to insulin. Once women reach the age of 50, they are more likely to gain visceral fat around their waist. This is a dangerous form of fat to carry around as it burdens the organs and puts

additional strain on the heart. As intermittent fasting is a highly sustainable way to shed this extra weight, it serves as a helping aid to improve heart health in this regard, too.

DIFFERENT TYPES OF INTERMITTENT FASTING TO CONSIDER BEYOND YOUR 50S

Once again, if this serves as your introduction to intermittent fasting, I strongly recommend that you opt for the 16/8 intermittent fasting method. Ease into it slowly and first aim for only 12/12 and then gradually move to the point where you can fast for 16 hours and limit eating to only eight hours per day.

The 5/2 method can also be highly effective for this age group as it doesn't require any days where you have to go without food. During the 5/2 method, you will eat five days as you would normally do and during the two remaining days, limit your food intake to account for only 500 calories. When you would like to have these two days during your week is completely up to you, and while you might enjoy greater benefits when you schedule these two days back-to-back, it is not necessary at all.

The more advanced version of the same eating style would be alternate-day fasting. As this will require that you count your calories every second day and eat far fewer calories during an entire week, you will see more rapid results from this way of eating. If this sounds like the solution that suits your lifestyle and your unique needs, then I recommend you start with the 5/2 method and gradually move into the alternate-day fasting method.

One reason why both these options are popular amongst more mature women is that you can still eat something vital, especially if you are on chronic medication and have to take your prescription at certain times. Having to take medicine three times per day during an eight-hour cycle of eating as per the 16/8 method might be challenging, while the 5/2 method restricts your calories and not your eating times.

Juice Fasting for Women of 50 and Beyond

While it may be the case that your health has deteriorated quite a bit by the time you are 50, many women are still extremely fit and active by the time they reach this milestone in their lives. Thus, depending on your overall health, you can opt for juice fasting to

increase weight loss. As you will only be consuming freshly pressed juice from fruit and vegetables with no additives or even fiber, your body won't be busy with digestion, and this frees your resources to take care of cell renewal and healing inside the body.

Don't juice fast for more than 72 hours, and return to either 5/2 fasting or 16/8 fasting to ensure that you keep off the weight you will lose during this phase.

The Pros and Cons of Water Fasting Beyond 50

Water fasting refers to a period during which you won't consume any calories and only hydrate your body with water. This way of fasting brings about many benefits and provides the body time to work through excess energy stored as fat, direct all bodily functions to heal and get rid of toxins, increase cell renewal and slow down the process of aging. I suggest that you never do a water fast for longer than 24 hours. If this is something that you do want to pursue, please discuss it with your medical professional first. Only you are aware of the overall state of your body, and it is best to gather professional advice before choosing such a radical form of fasting.

I don't recommend that you consider water fasting if you are on chronic medication or are suffering from any kind of health concern and haven't discussed your plans with your doctor first.

If you start to experience any side effects from not eating, like having headaches, feeling dizzy, light-headed, or fatigued, I do recommend that you stop immediately and first clear your health with your doctor before proceeding.

Is Dry Fasting Safe?

Dry fasting refers to a period during which you will consume nothing. You may not even drink any water during this rather radical form of fasting. Dry fasting might appear to be a solution to achieve weight loss, slow down the process of aging, and clear any inflammation, but it also has several risks linked to it.

Some risks linked to dry fasting include:

- Seizures because of a lack of necessary electrolytes in the body. When your body's level of electrolytes is out of sync, it negatively affects the signals between cells, and this can cause involuntary muscle contractions and seizures (Brennan, 2021a).
- When you re-introduce fluids after a dry fast, your body can absorb too much fluid, and this can cause brain swelling.
- Kidney failure is another concern to watch out for, as your body releases more toxins than usual during this fasting phase and, as you aren't taking in any fluid, your kidneys can get overloaded.
- Hypovolemic shock is the medical term for when your blood volume drops to a level where it affects your blood pressure and influences the level of oxygen available to your cells.
- These symptoms hold the potential to become quite severe and result in a coma or even death.

So, I don't recommend dry fasting for people above the age of 50, especially if they haven't followed a fasting regime until now.

WEIGHT LOSS BEYOND 50

There are several contributing factors to why weight loss is so much harder once you are older than 50.

Muscle Loss

Muscles require energy to sustain them, and when you lose muscle mass, your body requires fewer calories to function optimally. If you are not lowering your calorie intake, excess calories will be stored as fat, not only making it harder to lose weight but also to not gain weight. According to the American College of Sports Medicine, by the age of 50, we've lost about 10% of our muscle mass (Goad, 2021). While exercise can combat this, you also need to lower your calorie intake. It is why intermittent fasting options such as the 16/8 method can work wonders to reduce the number of calories you consume while preserving your muscle mass.

Slowing Down of the Metabolic Rate

Several contributing factors cause the metabolic rate to slow down after the age of 50. This means that you will also need less energy, as the physical processes taking place in the body are taking place at a much slower rate, and more calories are stored as fat cells rather than being used for energy.

Hormonal Changes

This is the time when most women start to experience menopause and the hormonal changes that take place in this phase of a woman's life. The production of estrogen is slowing down, making the body less sensitive to insulin, resulting in weight gain around the hips and waistline (Goad, 2021).

Being Less Active

While we desire to remain as active as we've always been, often, during this phase of your life, you begin to take things a little slower and become less active. It means that you need less energy but don't necessarily consume fewer calories. Excess calories always turn into fat.

However, while it might be more challenging to shed the extra weight after 50, it is possible, and many women have lost a significant amount of weight through intermittent fasting after turning 50 or even at a much more mature age.

Start with a short-term intermittent fasting method that best suits your lifestyle and explore how you lose not only weight but also begin to enjoy a range of other health benefits that go along with limiting your calorie intake and providing your body with a time when it doesn't have to digest food.

Once your body's resources are freed from digestion, it can attend to cell renewal, which aids in slowing down aging. I've also already discussed previously the many other health benefits you can enjoy from lowering the glucose levels in your bloodstream and using fat cells that are turned into ketones as an energy source rather than relying on glucose from eating with no limitations.

INTERMITTENT FASTING AND DIABETES FOR WOMEN ABOVE 50

It is estimated that about a third of the global population older than 65 years has diabetes (Diabetes and Older Adults, 2022). While this is already enough cause for concern, the even bigger concern is that people in this age group are much more prone to suffering from complications related to their diabetes. These complications can include hypoglycemia, heart disease, and kidney failure. While there is a range of treatment options available that will help you manage your diabetes effectively regardless of age, it is always preferred to prevent diabetes or to try to reverse the impact of the health concern.

While many studies have explored using intermittent fasting as a way to reverse the effect of diabetes, there is no conclusive evidence yet that intermittent fasting above 50 or any other age can be a miracle cure. Yet, several studies do indicate that intermittent fasting brings about several benefits that prevent not only diabetes—especially type 2 diabetes, which is often only diagnosed at a much more mature age— from developing. In certain cases, it can even reduce the impact of diabetes and improve overall health.

The fasting methods widely promoted as the most effective and safe ways for older adults to follow are the 16/8 method, 5/2 method, or alternate-day fasting. These methods bring about several health improvements, of which weight loss and lower glucose levels in the bloodstream are the most beneficial.

There are two points that I need to highlight if a diabetes prognosis serves as your inspiration to try intermittent fasting. Always make sure to enter this journey with the guidance of your health practitioner. When you are receiving treatment to manage your diabetes, it is most likely that your prescription is determined according to your usual eating habits. When you are changing this by fasting for several hours a day, your physician must change your prescription too.

The second point is that you need to start slowly. Any major disruptions can cause more harm than good. My suggestion would be that you start with the 5/2 approach and gradually move to reduce your calorie intake to where you only consume 500 or fewer calories on your two fasting days. Once your body has adjusted to this way of eating, you can increase your fasting days until you are at the point where you can comfortably implement alternate-day fasting.

In case you prefer the 16/8 method, start with 12/12 hours first. Gradually decrease your eating window until you are at 16/8.

If you are feeling any unpleasant symptoms from making these changes, reach out to your medical professional immediately.

Intermittent fasting does show promising results in diabetes treatment, and it can be a completely safe way to reduce the treatment your body requires and stop your diabetes from getting worse, but doing so responsibly is the key to your success.

Make sure that you monitor your blood sugar levels throughout so that you can act timeously if necessary.

The process also requires that you become more mindful and remain aware of any mood changes that might occur or if you experience fluctuations in your energy levels. It might even help to keep a journal to record any changes, which will make it easier to notice a pattern.

An important point to remember is not to flood your body with glucose during the times when you are eating. This will cause a spike in your glucose levels. The best way to address any foods that are high in carbohydrates is to limit them, and when you eat thesefoods, do so coupled with protein-rich food sources and vegetables rich in fiber.

FASTING TO LOOK YOUNGER

Once wrinkles start to show their presence on your skin, it is impossible to remove them completely. Yet, it is not too late to slow down the process of aging. Regardless of your age, beauty increases your level of confidence, and self-care is an act that makes you feel valued and is a way to show appreciation for your body.

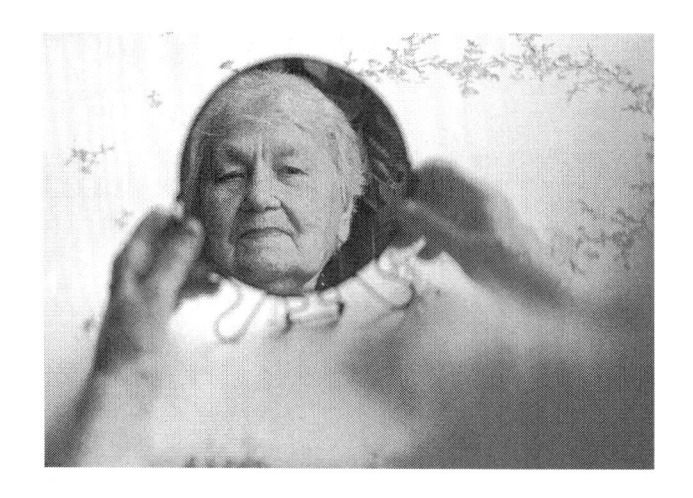

Thus, at this age, it is beneficial to consider intermittent fasting as a self-care routine that provides you with many reasons to feel confident, even if you are past the age of flaunting a young appearance. Now is the time to value your wisdom, traits, and experience and to live a full life. While you can enjoy all these emotional benefits from eating this way, you will also slow down the aging process, as intermittent fasting is linked to increased cell renewal and allows the body to get rid of dead skin cells and toxins that can make your skin look dull and tired much quicker.

While you might not be the spitting image of youth anymore, beauty is present in all ages. By looking your best and putting in time and effort i n t o your appearance and overall health, you will shave years off your age.

INTERMITTENT FASTING AND MEDICATION

The older we become, the more likely we are to have some prescription for chronic medication. For example, suppose you are a woman older than 50 who must take chronic medication. In that case, you can opt for intermittent fasting to improve your overall well-being.

Before just jumping into intermittent fasting, it is important to consider the bigger picture necessary to support a holistic approach to your well-being. Even following an intermittent fasting regime, there is enough time in your eating window to take your medicine. Still, you must be aware of how this way of eating might affect your medication regimen.

Intermittent fasting impacts how effective your prescription is. This can be for medication or supplements that you are taking. Fasting can have one of two outcomes. It might increase the level of absorption of your medication or decrease it.

The other concern is that fasting can worsen certain side effects of the medicine. For example, say that the medication you are taking leaves you feeling a little nauseous after taking it; fasting might increase the level of nausea you are experiencing (Chan, 2021). Again, however, the effect that it will have differs from person to person, and the best advice is just to be aware of whether you are experiencing any of these concerns.

While saying that, simply by taking preventative steps, you can manage chronic medication well along with your new eating style. I am sharing some tips to serve as guidance on this journey.

Vitamins

When taking vitamins A, D, E, or K, it is important to know that these are all fat-soluble vitamins. Your digestive system will absorb them the best when you take them along with fatty foods. This doesn't mean that you need to eat food prepared in fat, but it helps to take them after a meal that includes healthy oils like nuts, avocados, fish, or seeds. Red meat is also high in fat and will aid in absorbing these vitamins too (Chan, 2021).

Iron Supplements

Iron supplements tend to cause digestive concerns, and intermittent fasting might improve the situation. While it will help to take your iron supplement with food, taking

it, along with citrus fruits or juices, will not only improve how your body absorbs iron butalso help reduce any digestive concerns it might cause (Chan, 2021).

Diabetes Medication

This is one of the chronic descriptions that you need to discuss with your doctor before starting intermittent fasting. Suppose you continue with your diabetes prescription and go through fasting. In that case, you might increase your risk of hypoglycemia, which presents symptoms like dizziness, fatigue, and even seizures if your blood sugar level is too lowfor too long (Chan, 2021).

Thyroid Medication

The biggest point of interest regarding thyroid medication is how your body absorbs it. Research indicates that during the fasting phase, the absorption rate of thyroid medication is as high as 80% and drops to 60% when taking it after a meal. So, for the best results, it might be best to take your thyroid medication about half an hour before breaking your fast. Yet, here, too, it is best to determine the optimal timing for yourneeds with the help of your doctor.

Most Over-the-Counter Medicine

When you are taking over-the-counter medicine, it is more than likely that it is some version of pain medication like ibuprofen. However, these medicines shouldn't be taken on an empty stomach, as this can cause various medical concerns like heartburn, constipation, stomach pain, and nausea. Rather, wait until you are in your eating window and have them either with your meal or a glass of milk (Chan, 2021).

Can Medication Break My Fast?

The shortest answer to this is yes. It is even more so when the medication you are taking contains sugar. Many multivitamins are available today in the form of gummies, and these always contain sugar or some kind of sweetener. However, these aren't the only types of medication or supplements that contain sugar. Some pills have a sugar coating around them, which can be enough sugar to trigger your glucose levels to the degree that breaks your fast. So, it is best to always wait for your eating window if you can.

While this might sound complex, it doesn't have to be, and you only need to ensure that you are getting your timing exactly right for your needs. Again, there is no better person toprovide you with exact instructions on this than your doctor.

8

RECIPES

No one is born a great cook; one learns by doing.

— JULIA CHILD

You know now when to eat and when to fast. Now it is time to explore the meals that will help you optimize your weight loss during your eating window. I am sharing ten recipes that are low in calories and high in nutrients and that will help to make your life much easier. I also want to urge you to experiment a bit in the kitchen. Try different versions of these recipes and claim your healthy lifestyle.

BLUEBERRY GRANOLA TREAT

Crispy and fruity and simply divine. It is a delicious treat that is low in calories and filled with fiber. I hope you enjoy it as much as I do.

Time: 50 minutes

Serving Size: 6

Prep Time: 5 minutes

Cook Time: 45 minutes

Nutritional Facts/Info:

Calories: 395

Carbs: 119.5 g

Fat: 1.6 g

Protein: 19.4 g

Ingredients:

- 16 oz bag of blueberries
- 8 oz box of sugar-free vanilla pudding mix
- ¼ cup nonfat milk
- ½ tsp nutmeg
- 1 tsp cinnamon
- 1 ½ cup oats
- 8 oz plain, fat-free yogurt

- ½ cup sugar substitute
- 1 tsp almond extract

Directions:

1. Preheat the oven to 350°F.
2. Prepare an 8 x 8-inch baking pan by coating it with a thin layer of oil.
3. Use the baking pan to mix the blueberries, pudding mix, non-fat milk, nutmeg, and cinnamon.
4. Combine the oats, yogurt, sugar substitute, and almond extract, and spoon it over the berry mixture.
5. Bake for 45 minutes or until the top is golden brown and crunchy.

SPICY DAL FOR A COLD DAY

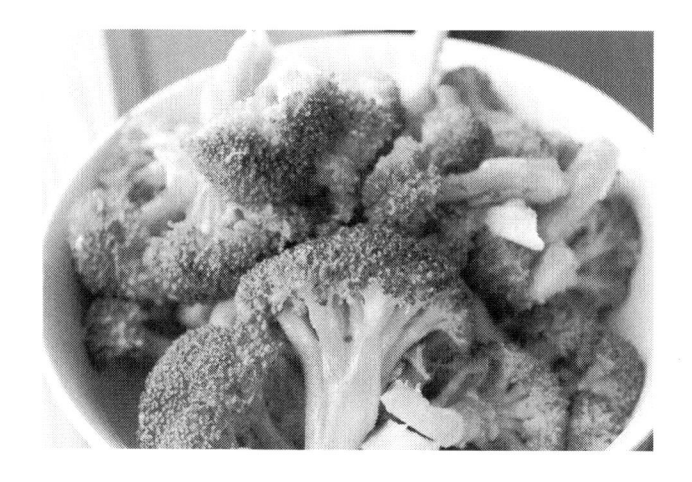

It is usually on days when it is cold outside that we crave all kinds of treats. Yes, I too love food—the flavors and the textures, but also the satisfaction you gain from a warm and tasty meal that just hit the perfect spot. This dal is for those days when you simply need something to help you warm up from the inside. Dal is a vegetarian curry that has lentils as the key ingredient. It takes a little longer to make, but it's worth every minute. This recipe is also quite lenient and can be the perfect option to experiment with by adding desired ingredients. I sometimes add fresh chili to spice it up even more.

Time: 1 hour 30 minutes

Serving Size: 4

Prep Time: 25 minutes

Cook Time: 1 hour 5 minutes

Nutritional Facts/Info:

Calories: 711

Carbs: 89.9 g

Fat: 34.3 g

Protein: 27.3 g

Ingredients:

- 4 tbsp butter or ghee
- 2 onions, chopped
- 1 tsp chili powder
- 2 tsp cumin
- 1 1/2 tsp black pepper
- 2 tsp turmeric
- 1 tsp ground coriander
- 1 cup red lentil
- Juice of 1 lemon
- 3 cups chicken broth
- 2 broccoli heads, chopped
- 1/2 cup dried coconut (optional)
- 1 tbsp flour
- 1 tsp salt
- 1 cup cashews, coarsely chopped (optional)

Directions:

1. Heat a medium-sized saucepan and sauté the onion in the butter until it turns brown.
2. Mix in the chili powder, cumin, black pepper, turmeric, and coriander, and fry for about a minute while stirring.
3. Add in the lentils, lemon juice, and broth. If you are using coconut, you can add this too. While the coconut is optional, it adds extra fullness and flavor to the meal.
4. Use high heat to bring the saucepan to boil and then reduce the heat to let the mixture simmer for about 55 minutes. You want the lentils to be soft. Stir occasionally to prevent the mixture from burning; if it is too thick, you can add a little water.
5. Bring another pot with water to boil. Add your broccoli pieces, and once the water boils again, remove the broccoli and place it in a bowl of cold water to stop the cooking process.
6. Take a few spoons of the lentil mixture and combine it with the flour in a separate bowl. Once it has formed a paste, you can add it to the saucepan again and stir it in. Let the pot simmer for about 5 minutes to allow the sauce to thicken. If you have a blending stick, you can also give the pot of lentils a quick whizz to ensure a smoother texture.
7. Add salt to taste.

8. Add the broccoli and let it simmer for another 5 minutes.
9. Serve with basmati rice and sprinkle some nuts on top if you prefer.

PIZZA THE HEALTHY WAY

Pizza is a winner every time and can be the perfect meal on the go or as comfort food. It is also hard to beat leftover pizza when you can have it the next day. Yet, it is usually a meal that is burdened with calories, as the base is loaded with carbs and the toppings we choose. In this recipe, we replace the base with cauliflower, which is far less calorie-dense and high in fiber. This is a trusted recipe enticing even my friends, who don't like cauliflower, to return for more.

Time: 1 hour 10 minutes

Serving Size: 4

Prep Time: 20 minutes

Cook Time: 50 minutes

Nutritional Facts/Info:

Calories: 198

Carbs: 7 g

Fat: 12.9 g

Protein: 12.8 g

Ingredients:

- 4 cups cauliflower rice
- 1 egg
- 1 cup soft cheese
- 1 tsp oregano
- Salt to taste

Directions:

1. Heat the oven to 400°F.
2. You can buy cauliflower rice already made, but if you can't find it, another (much more affordable) option is to wash your cauliflower head and chop it into smaller chunks. Then you can blend it until it has a texture similar to rice.
3. Fill a large pot with about an inch of water and bring it to a boil. Add the cauliflower rice and let it cook for only 5 minutes. Then strain the water with a fine-mesh sieve.

4. The next step is vital to your success. It is important to dry the rice as much as possible, so once you've strained the water, transfer the rice to a clean dishcloth. Let it cool down for a bit before wrapping it in the dishcloth and squeezing all the water out of the rice. Preferably work over a basin, as this can get messy. Squeeze as much as you can to dry out the rice as much as you can.
5. Once dry, you can place the rice in a large mixing bowl.
6. Beat the egg slightly and then add it along with the soft cheese and spices to the rice.
7. Prepare a baking sheet with parchment paper.
8. Mix it all. I've found that using my hands works best. If this doesn't look like pizza dough, don't be too concerned. The final product makes up for it all.
9. Place the cauliflower dough on the prepared baking sheet and press it down to form the crust of your pizza. The thinner you make the crust, the crispier the end product.
10. Bake the crust for about 40 minutes until it is firm and golden brown.
11. Remove from the oven and add your favorite pizza toppings. You are free to choose any options you like, but remember that even with pizza toppings, there are healthier choices that you can make. I like mushrooms, olives, and not too much cheese, as cheese is so high in calories.

12. Return to the hot oven and bake for another 10 minutes until the topping bubbles.

HEALTHY BURRITOS

You might notice that I want to show you that even when you opt for healthier alternatives, you can still indulge in the most widely enjoyed favorites. These burritos offer so much more than a calorie-rich snack as the ingredients are also full of nutrients. This is a meal that feeds the body and the soul.

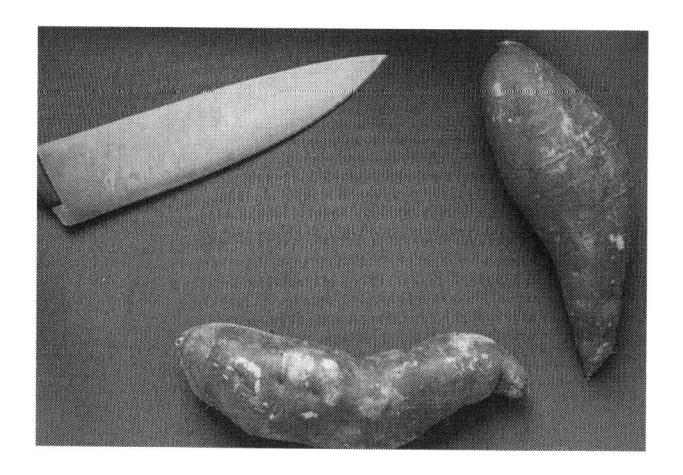

Time: 1 hour 5 minutes

Serving Size: 10

Prep Time: 15 minutes

Cook Time: 50 minutes

Nutritional Facts/Info:

Calories: 466

Carbs: 105.9 g

Fat: 3.5 g

Protein: 23.9 g

Ingredients:

- 5 cups sweet potatoes, peeled and cubed
- 1/2 tsp salt
- 2 tsp vegetable oil
- 3 1/2 cups onions, diced
- 1 tbsp fresh green chili pepper, minced
- Four garlic cloves, minced
- 4 tsp coriander
- 4 tsp cumin
- 4 1/2 cups black beans, cooked and drained
- 2/3 cup cilantro leaves, chopped
- 2 tbsp lemon juice
- Salt to taste
- 12 flour tortillas
- Fresh salsa

Directions:

1. Heat the oven to 350°F.
2. Prepare a large baking dish with a thin layer of oil.

3. Use a medium-sized saucepan, add water, sweet potatoes, and salt, and bring it to boil on high heat. Once it boils, reduce the heat and let it simmer for about 10 minutes. Then drain the sweet potato and set it aside.
4. Sauté the onions, chili, and garlic in the oil in a medium skillet. After about 7 minutes, the onions should be soft, and you can add coriander and cumin. Let it cook for 3 minutes while constantly stirring to prevent burning.
5. Use a food processor to blend the black beans, cilantro, lemon juice, and sweet potatoes. Salt to taste. If you don't have a blender, you can also mash it by hand in a large bowl.
6. Add the onion and spice mixture.
7. Divide the mixture between the number of tortillas you have and spoon the mixture into the center of each tortilla. Roll your tortillas and place them seam down in the baking dish.
8. Cover the dish with foil and bake for roughly 30 minutes until the tortillas are hot.
9. Remove from the oven and serve with fresh salsa.

MILLET AND QUINOA–TASTY AND HEALTHY

Once you become more comfortable with this healthier way of eating, you can find new and different foods that are far tastier than processed foods and way healthier. Two grains that are not used in recipes enough are millet and quinoa. Quinoa is the seeds of the flowering plant that contain high levels of protein, fiber, and B vitamins. Millet is also a seed, and, while not as high in proteins, it still contains a fairly decent amount of protein for a grain. In addition, it is high in fiber and an excellent replacement for other grains like white rice. This salad stays perfect for about two days if you keep it in the refrigerator.

Time: 40 minutes

Serving Size: 4

Prep Time: 15 minutes

Cook Time: 25 minutes

Nutritional Facts/Info:

Calories: 574

Carbs: 91.2 g

Fat: 12.5 g

Protein: 27.8 g

Ingredients:

- 1/2 cup millet
- 1 cup water
- 1/2 cup quinoa
- 3/4 cup water

- 1 English cucumber, diced
- 1 tomato, seeds squeezed out, diced
- 1 sweet pepper, seeded and diced
- 1/2 red onion, sliced thin
- 1 garlic clove, pressed
- 200 g feta cheese, diced
- 10 oz can of white beans, drained
- Cayenne pepper to taste
- 2 tsp dried dill
- 1/4 cup pine nuts
- Juice of 1 lemon (zest as well, if preferred)
- 1 tbsp olive oil (optional)
- Black pepper to taste

Directions:

1. Use a medium-sized pot and bring the millet and 1 cup of water to boil. Let it simmer on lower heat for about 10 minutes with the lid on. Once cooked, you can drain any excess water if any is left. Then, let it cool down to room temperature.
2. In a second pot, bring the quinoa and ¾ cup of water to boil. Let it simmer on lower heat with the lid on for about 15 minutes and when the water is cooked dry, fluff the quinoa with a fork. Let it cool down to room temperature.
3. Use a large mixing bowl and combine all the ingredients.

4. Mix well and let it chill for about an hour before serving.

BLACK-EYED PEAS FOR A SLOW DAY

As a woman, you have many roles to fill. This can be challenging and exhausting. However, it also means that some days there is little time to prepare food, and other days you have far more time for cooking. This recipe is perfect for those days when you can take things a little slower.

Time: 10 hours 5 minutes

Serving Size: 6

Prep Time: 5 minutes

Cook Time: 10 hours

Nutritional Facts/Info:

Calories: 329

Carbs: 12 g

Fat: 13.8 g

Protein: 38.1 g

Ingredients:

- 16 oz dried black-eyed peas
- 1 small ham hock

- 14 oz can of jalapeno peppers
- 14 oz can of tomatoes diced with green chilies
- 20 oz can of chicken broth
- 1 stalk celery, chopped

Directions:

1. Soak the black-eyed peas overnight in water.
2. Drain the water from the beans and add all the ingredients to a slow cooker.
3. Cook for about 10 hours until all ingredients are soft and tasty.

SALTY AND SATISFYING OATS BOWL

Sure, we are all familiar with oats cooked the normal way—I mean, of course, with sugar and maybe a dash of milk. But as oats are a grain, like rice or even couscous, you can also turn oats into a savory meal. This recipe might initially sound a little unusual, but just try it once, and you'll see how you can transform oats into something completely different.

Time: 40 minutes

Serving Size: 4

Prep Time: 10 minutes

Cook Time: 30 minutes

Nutritional Facts/Info:

Calories: 460

Carbs: 56.7 g

Fat: 16.9 g

Protein: 19.9 g

Ingredients:

- 16 oz bag of cubed butternut squash
- 8 oz Brussels sprouts, halved
- 1 tbsp olive oil
- 1 tsp salt
- 1 tsp black pepper
- 1 tbsp butter
- ½ cup onion, coarsely chopped
- 2 cups oats
- 2 cup water
- ½ cup cheddar cheese, shredded
- 4 eggs
- 2 strips cooked turkey bacon, crumbled

Directions:

1. Prepare a large baking sheet with parchment paper and heat the oven to 400°F.
2. Use a large bowl to combine the Brussels sprouts, butternut, onion, salt and pepper, and olive oil.

3. Roast this in the oven for about 20 minutes. The vegetables must be soft and golden brown but not overcooked. I get the best results if I roast my vegetables high-up in the oven, almost right underneath the grill section.
4. Use a medium-sized pot to melt the butter and add the oats. Stir until the oats have a toasted color and flavor. Then add the water and bring it to a boil. Reduce the heat and let it simmer for about 10 minutes.
5. Stir in the shredded cheese and season to taste with salt and pepper.
6. Cook the eggs according to your preference.
7. Use four bowls to scoop in the oats and top it off with the roasted vegetables and egg. Finally, sprinkle some of the turkey bacon crumbles over for added flavor.
8. This is also one of those recipes where you can easily add some personal flair with additional ingredients. For example, why not try the oats with olives or roasted tomatoes and maybe just a light sprinkle of chopped chili.

BONE BROTH

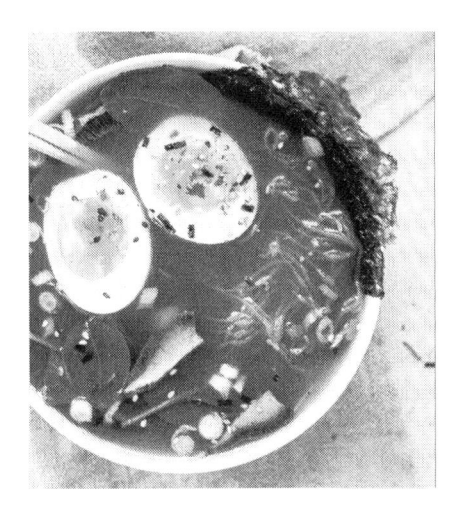

A list of the most valuable recipes to benefit your overall health and well-being would not be complete without a bone broth recipe. This is the type of dish that is very versatile, as you can add vegetables, ramen noodles, or even a poached egg to make it a

more substantial meal. As it is jam-packed with nutrition, it is a meal that brings so many benefits to the table. I like to use oxtail for my bone broth, as I know this is the meat of excellent quality, but you can also opt to use meaty bones. Ultimately, the bone is the star of this recipe, and the meat on the outside is merely for added flavor. Sometimes, I don't even strain my broth as I enjoy it as a soup that still contains all the chunky parts.

The benefits of bone broth are:

- It improves digestion as it supports gut health, affecting your entire system.
- Bone broth is a rich source of collagen and is, therefore, a vital role player in theprocess of slowing down aging.
- The collagen content also supports joint health.
- Some studies show that bone broth is important in immune support asit is nutrient-dense.
- Bone broth contains the amino acid glycine, which plays a supporting role in ensuring healthy sleeping habits.

Time: 9 hours 30 minutes

Serving Size: 4

Prep Time: 30 minutes

Cook Time: 9 hours

Nutritional Facts/Info:

Calories: 167

Carbs: 6.3 g

Fat: 7.6 g

Protein: 18.3 g

Ingredients:

- 4 lbs oxtail
- 2 unpeeled carrots, cut into 2-inch pieces
- 1 leek, ends trimmed, cut into 2-inch pieces
- 1 onion, quartered
- 1 garlic head, halved crosswise
- 2 celery stalks, cut into 2-inch pieces
- 2 bay leaves
- 2 tbsp black peppercorns
- 1 tbsp cider vinegar

Directions:

1. Heat the oven to 450°F.
2. Use a large baking tray and heat the tray up in the oven until it is piping hot.
3. Remove the tray from the oven and place the oxtail, vegetables, and garlic in the baking tray and roast it all until it has a rich brown color. This will take about 40 minutes. You can turn the pieces of oxtail over halfway through the baking time.
4. Use a large stockpot and add 12 cups of water. Add the celery, bay leaves, peppercorns, and vinegar to the pot. Now add the browned vegetables and oxtail. Ensure all the juice from the meat and vegetables also goes into the pot.

5. You can add more water if all the bones and vegetables aren't covered.
6. Bring the pot to a boil. Then place the lid on the pot, but make sure that it is ajar so that the steam from the pot can escape. Again, you want the fluid to reduce.
7. Leave the pot to simmer on low heat for at least 8 hours and as long as 24 hours. Then, at night, simply turn off the pot and turn it back on the next morning to continue the cooking process. The secret to bone broth is that the longer it is simmering, the better it becomes.
8. Just take care to check in on your pot at intervals and if you see any foam on top, scoop it off with a spoon.
9. Once you are done cooking the bone broth, let it cool down to room temperature. Then you can remove the bones and strain out any solid parts that are left over from the vegetables. You can use a sieve for this.
10. Pour the bone broth into portion-sized containers and place them in the refrigerator. When the broth has cooled down completely, scoop off the solidified fat on top.
11. When you are ready to eat your bone broth, simply reheat and enjoy. Bone broth stays good for about five days in the refrigerator, and you can freeze it for as long assix months.

A FINAL WORD

What I want to achieve with these recipes is to show that while you can eat anything you like during the window when you can, it will be to your benefit to not indulge solely in unhealthy foods. When you transition to intermittent fasting and make this your new way of living, you do so to ensure lasting good health and vitality, and it will only benefit you to eat foods that support this cause.

The recipes I've shared are also far from being the only healthy and tasty meals you can indulge in. I want you to try out different dishes and see how you can add variation to these meals. Use the time of transition to change your relationship with food. Notice flavors, what works well together, and which flavors you enjoy. By eating slowly, you will start to enjoy your food. This is when the mind shift takes place between living to eat and eating to live. Bon appétit!

BEFORE YOU FINISH THIS BOOK...

Grab Your Free Book Triple Fasting

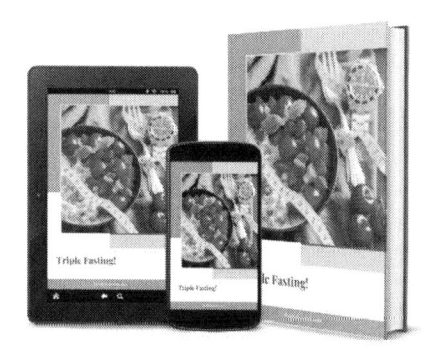

IN HERE YOU WILL LEARN:

3 Key Secrets You **MUST DO** Before Starting Your Intermittent Fasting Journey!

Scan the QR code:

CONCLUSION

Whether you are 20, 40, or even 60, it is never too late to start with intermittent fasting and unleash the many benefits it holds. It is a way of eating that dates back very far into history, a way of eating that is far healthier than our modern-day diet. It is also a way of eating that can reverse several of the negative effects modern-day living has on our physical, mental, and emotional health and well-being.

It is a way of eating that is sustainable and adaptable to suit your lifestyle. It is adjustable, so at times you can be stricter, and you can have a more relaxed approach to your fasting windows. Intermittent fasting doesn't prohibit you from eating anything you like. When you crave something, you will only have to wait a few hours at most before you can indulge a little.

That said, it will be beneficial to maintain a healthy eating plan during your eating windows if you want to see rapid results and gain as much out of this lifestyle as it offers. It is also a way of losing weight and improving your well-being even if you are battling several health concerns. Still, if you do, I want to urge you to discuss your eating strategy with your doctor first. While intermittent fasting is safe and effective, it might not be the best solution for you, or maybe you need to change to accommodate your unique needs in your eating plan.

Suppose you have been struggling with weight all your life and have been trying so many fad diets that you've lost count along the way. In that case, I want you to try intermittent fasting rather than giving up hope on a future where you can live a fulfilled and healthy life. In this book, I've provided you with all the tools you need to get started on this journey, and I hope that in a year from now, you too can look back, just like my best friend, and know that this was the best choice that you've made for yourself.

Take care of yourself and your physical, mental, and emotional health, not because you have to, but because you deserve nothing less. Transform your eating habits from a routine that leaves you feeling weak and ashamed into a tool that empowers you to achieve much more in life, in all the arenas where success is waiting.

Proceed with caution and reap the benefits waiting for you. If you enjoyed this book, please leave a review on Amazon.

BIBLIOGRAPHY

Boone, R. (2014, December 30). *Beef bone broth*. Epicurious. https://www.epicurious.com/recipes/food/views/beef-bone-broth-51260700

Boyers, L. (2020, February 21). *Is intermittent fasting safe for women? All your questions answered*. Mindbodygreen. https://www.mindbodygreen.com/articles/guide-to-healthy-intermittent-fasting-for-women/

Cahn, L. (2022, March 7). *16 Self-care quotes that will inspire you to care for your mind and body*. The Healthy. https://www.thehealthy.com/mental-health/self-care/self-care-quotes/

Canyon Ranch. (2021, Aug 14). *How women's bodies change with age: 30, 40, 50 & beyond*. WellStated. https://www.canyonranch.com/well-stated/post/a-womans-changing-body/

Chan, T. (2021, January 4). *Does taking medication break intermittent fasting?* Simple. https://simple.life/blog/intermittent-fasting-and-medication/

Cherry, K. (2022, January 26). *How to improve your self-control*. Verywell Mind. https://www.verywellmind.com/psychology-of-self-control-4177125

Davids Landau, M. (2022, January). *Intermittent fasting around menopause: does it make sense?* EverydayHealth. https://www.everydayhealth.com/womens-health/what-midlife-women-should-know-about-intermittent-fasting/

Davis, C. P. (2021, March). *How long do you need to fast for autophagy?* MedicineNet.https://www.medicinenet.com/how_long_do_you_need_to_-fast_for_autophagy/article.htm

Diabetesandolderadults.(2022,January).Endocrine. https://www.endocrine.org/patient-engagement/endocrine-library/diabetes-and-olderadults#:~:text=An%20estimated%2033%25%20of%20adults

Ellis, S. (2017, March 10). *How should you exercise while you're intermittent Fasting?*Mindbodygreen.https://www.mindbodygreen.com/0-29179/how-should-you-exercise-while-youre-intermittent-fasting-doctors-weigh-in.html

Fasting can slow down aging! (2020, January). The Times of India. https://timesofindia.indiatimes.com/life-style/food-news/can-fasting-slow-down-aging/articleshow/73067733.cms

Felson,S.(2020,June).*Livewellover50.*WebMD. https://www.webmd.com/healthy-aging/ss/slideshow-live-well-over-50#:~:text=Changing%20your%20lifestyle%20in%20you

4 tricks to stick to intermittent fasting easily. (2019, September). Times of India. https://timesofindia.indiatimes.com/life-style/health-fitness/diet/4-tricks-to-stick-to-intermittent-fasting-easily/articleshow/70978326.cms?

Fuentes, L. S. (2018, December 6). *Roasted veggie and savory oats bowl.* Laura Fuentes. https://www.laurafuentes.com/roasted-veggies-savory-oats-bowl/

Goad, K. (2021, June). *5 Factors that make weight loss harder after 50.* AARP. https://www.aarp.org/health/healthy-living/info-2021/weight-loss-after-50.html#:~:text=By%20age%2050%2C%20you

Goerl, B. (2021, June 21). To skip or not to skip: Does intermittent fasting help peoplewithdiabetes?DiaTribe. https://diatribe.org/skip-or-not-skip-does-intermittent-fasting-help-people-diabetes

Gunnars, K. (2016, August 16). *10 Evidence-based health benefits of intermittent fasting.*Healthline. https://www.healthline.com/nutrition/10-health-benefits-of-intermittent-fasting

Gunnars, K. (2020a, April 20). *Intermittent fasting 101—The ultimate beginner's guide.*Healthline.https://www.healthline.com/nutrition/intermittent-fasting-guide

Gunnars, K. (2020b, September 25). *How Intermittent Fasting Can Help You LoseWeight.*Healthline. https://www.healthline.com/nutrition/intermittent-fasting-and-weight-loss#fasting-plans

Hatanaka, M. (2020, June 11). *Intermittent fasting and exercise: How to do it safely.*MedicalNewsToday. https://www.medicalnewstoday.com/articles/intermittent-fasting-and-working-out#safety-tips

Heshmat, S. (2017, March). *10 Strategies for developing self-control.* Psychology Today.https://www.psychologytoday.com/za/blog/science-choice/201703/10-strategies-developing-self-control

HGH & Intermittent fasting: Can fasting increase HGH? (2021, October 21). 21 Day Hero. https://21dayhero.com/hgh-intermittent-fasting/

Hodgson, L. (2021, March 31). *Intermittent fasting with diabetes: A Guide.* Healthline.https://www.healthline.com/health/type-2-diabetes/intermittent-fasting-and-diabetes-safe

How to make intermittent fasting work for you. (2020, October). Vault. https://www.vaulthealth.com/blog/articles/how-to-make-intermittent-fasting-work-for-you

Intermittent fasting. (n.d.). Pinterest. https://za.pinterest.com/drannayoung/intermittent-fasting/

Intermittent fasting benefits for seniors. (n.d.). Visiting Angels. https://www.visitingangels.com/jenkintown/articles/intermittent-fasting-benefits-for-seniors/18643

Intermittent fasting: What is it, and how does it work? (2021). Johns Hopkins Medicine. https://www.hopkinsmedicine.org/health/wellness-and-prevention/intermittent-fasting-what-is-it-and-how-does-it-work

Jacobs, R. (2019, December 27). *How changing your mindset can radically transform your eating habits.* FitOn - #1 Free Fitness App, Stop Paying for Home Workouts. https://fitonapp.com/wellness/transform-eating-habits/

Jelinek, J. (2021, July 29). *Ways to change habits.* PsychCentral. https://psychcentral.com/health/steps-to-changing-a-bad-habit#recap

Jim Rohn Quotes. (n.d.). BrainyQuote. https://www.brainyquote.com/quotes/jim_rohn_109882

Kidadle Team. (2022, May). *70+ Skin care quotes to help you look after your body.* Kidadl. https://kidadl.com/quotes/skin-care-quotes-to-help-you-look-after-your-body

Kucine, J. (2018, November 8). *Benefits of intermittent fasting.* Dr. Jeff Kucine D.O. https://www.drkucine.com/benefits-of-intermittent-fasting/

Leiva, C. (2018, October). *The best and worst types of intermittent fasting, according to experts.* Insider. https://www.insider.com/best-worst-intermittent-fasting-types-2018-9#overall-intermittent-fasting-can-be-good-for-your-gut-5

Leptin: What it is, function & levels. (n.d.). Cleveland Clinic. https://my.cleve landclinic.org/health/articles/22446-leptin#:~:text=Leptin

Lett, R. (2019, August 9). *7 Types of intermittent fasting, explained.* Span. https://www.span.health/blog/7-types-of-intermittent-fasting-explained

Levy, J. (2018, November 5). *Signs you need this vital enzyme & how to get it.* Dr. Axe. https://draxe.com/nutrition/pepsin/

Lindberg, S. (2020, September 1). *How to exercise safely during intermittent fasting.*Healthline.https://www.healthline.com/health/how-to-exercise-safely-intermittent-fasting

Link, R. (2018, July 30). *8 Health benefits of fasting, backed by science.*Healthline.https://www.healthline.com/nutrition/fasting-benefits#TOC_TI-TLE_HDR_9

MacMahan, D. (2020, September). *How intermittent fasting helped this woman loseweightduringquarantine.*TODAY. https://www.today.com/health/how-intermittent-fasting-during-quarantine-helped-one-woman-t192396

Mid-life crisis begins in mid-30s, Relate survey says. (2010, September 28). *BBC News.* https://www.bbc.com/news/health-11429993

Migala, J. (2020, April 20). *7 Types of intermittent fasting: which is best for you?* EverydayHealth https://www.everydayhealth.com/diet-nutrition/diet/types-intermittent-fasting-which-best-you/

National Institute of Diabetes and Digestive and Kidney Diseases. (2019, May 12). *Health risks of overweight & obesity.* National Institute of Diabetes and DigestiveandKidneyDiseases. https://www.niddk.nih.gov/health-information/weight-management/adult-overweight-obesity/health-risks

Ogłodek, E., & Pilis, Prof., W. (2021). Is water-only fasting safe? *Global Advances inHealthandMedicine,10,*216495612110311. https://doi.org/10.1177/21649561211031178

PictureQuotes.com.(n.d.).PictureQuotes http://www.picturequotes.com/even-a-woman-of-abnormal-will-cannot-escape-her-hormonal-identity-quote-299869

Pratt, E. (2020, May 15). *Processed foods: Health risks and what to avoid.* MedicalNewsToday. https://www.medicalnewstoday.com/articles/318630#is-it-bad-for-you

Publishing, H. H. (2020, April 1). *Is intermittent fasting safe for older adults?* HarvardHealth.https://www.health.harvard.edu/staying-healthy/is-intermittent-fasting-safe-for-older-adults

Putka, S. (n.d.). *Male and female bodies can respond differently to intermittent fasting.*Inverse.https://www.inverse.com/mind-body/intermittent-fasting-difference-men-women

Raman, R. (2017, September 24). *Why your metabolism slows down with age.* Healthline. https://www.healthline.com/nutrition/metabolism-and-age

Revelant, J. (2021, October). *Is intermittent fasting safe for people with diabetes?*EverydayHealth https://www.everydayhealth.com/type-2-diabetes/diet/intermittent-fasting-safe-people-with-diabetes/

Roberts, C. (2021, May 24). *The different types of intermittent fasting.* HealthCentral. https://www.healthcentral.com/condition/intermittent-fasting-types

Rohn, J. (n.d.) "Take care of your body. It's the only place you have to live." Pass ItOn. https://www.passiton.com/inspirational-quotes/7279-take-care-of-your-body-its-the-only-place-you#:~:text=%E2%80%9CTake%20-

care%20of%20your%20body

RVS Chaitanya Koppala. (2017, March 3). *Gastrointestinal hormones (Gastrin, secretinandcholecystokinin)*.Slideshare. https://www.slideshare.net/ckoppala/gastrointestinal-hormones-gastrin-secretin-and-cholecystokinin

Schneider, J. (2020, October 7). *The healthy aging benefits of autophagy & how toactivatethecellularprocess*.Mindbodygreen. https://www.mindbodygreen.com/articles/autophagy/

Schneider, J. (2021, September 9). *The link between intermittent fasting & youthfulskin*.Mindbodygreen. https://www.mindbodygreen.com/articles/link-between-intermittent-fasting-and-youthful-skin/

7 Incredible things intermittent fasting does for your brain. (2020, March). AmenClinics. https://www.amenclinics.com/blog/7-incredible-things-intermittent-fasting-does-for-your-brain/#:~:text=Research%20in%20the%20Journal%20of

Shatzman, C. (2019, October 1). *Intermittent fasting is the only thing that stoppedmycramps*.SheKnows. https://www.sheknows.com/health-and-wellness/articles/2102543/intermittent-fasting-period-cramps/

Shiffer, E. (2021, May 6). *You need to see these jaw-dropping intermittent fastingweightlosstransformations*.Women'sHealth. https://www.womenshealthmag.com/weight-loss/g28836098/intermittent-fasting-before-and-after/

Sisson, M (n.d.). *How to exercise while fasting*. Mark's Daily Apple. https://www.marksdailyapple.com/how-to-exercise-while-fasting/#:~:text=The%20simplest%20form%20of%20exercise

Successstories.(n.d.).GinStephens,AuthorandIntermittentFaster. https://www.ginstephens.com/success-stories.html

The essential role of hormones in your daily functions: The well for health: Health and wellness center. (n.d.). Www.thewellforhealth.com. https://www.thewellforhealth.com/blog/the-essential-role-of-hormones-in-your-daily-functions

32Topintermittentfastingrecipes.(n.d.).Food. https://www.food.com/ideas/intermittent-fasting-recipes-6939

Thurrott, S. (2020, January). *How this woman used intermittent fasting to lose 80poundsinayear.*NBCNews. https://www.nbcnews.com/better/lifestyle/how-one-woman-used-intermittent-fasting-lose-80-pounds-year-ncna1124121

Tiger, L. (2021, February). *Quotes to make you feel better about getting older.* TheHealthy.https://www.thehealthy.com/aging/healthy-aging/quotes-about-getting-older/

Top25fastingquotes.(n.d.).A-ZQuotes. https://www.azquotes.com/quotes/topics/fasting.html

Type2diabetescausesandriskfactors.(n.d.).WebMD. https://www.webmd.com/diabetes/diabetes-causes

WebMD Editorial Contributors. (2021, April). *Is dry fasting safe?* WebMD. https://www.webmd.com/diet/is-dry-fasting-safe

WebMD Editorial Contributors. (2021, June). *What to know about juice fasting.* WebMD. https://www.webmd.com/diet/what-to-know-about-juice-fasting

WeCareBlog. (2021, July). *Intermittent fasting an effective way to manage type-1diabetes?*MedtronicDiabetes. https://www.medtronic-diabetes.com/en-ZA/blog/intermittent-fasting-effective-way-manage-type-1-diabetes-find-out-what-research-says#:~:text=Researchers%20have%20demonstrated%20that%20intermittent

Weight loss: Intermittent fasting tips for women above 40: Things to know. (2022,February9). TheTimesofIndia. https://timesofindia.indiatimes.com/life-style/health-fitness/diet/intermittent-f%20asting-tips-for-women-above-40-things-to-know/photostory/89373940.cms?pici%20d=89373948

West, H. (2021, July 19). *Does intermittent fasting boost your metabolism?* Healthline.https://www.healthline.com/nutrition/intermittent-fasting-metabolism#metabolism-boost

Wheatherspoon, D. (2019). *Midlife crisis in women: How it feels, what causes it, andwhattodo.*Healthline. https://www.healthline.com/health/midlife-crisis-women

Wilson, D. R. (2015, January 30). *Signs and symptoms of high estrogen: Diagnosis,treatment,andmore.*Healthline. https://www.healthline.com/health/high-estrogen#complications

IMAGE SOURCES

Andrade, F. (2020). *White powder on brown textile.* [Image]. Unsplash. https://unsplash.com/photos/sEi3apr6Vys

Bailey, J. (2018). *Flat lay photography of turned-on silver iPad besideApple.* [Image]. Unsplash. https://unsplash.com/photos/94Ld_MtIUf0

Carstens-Peters. G. (2017). *Chocolate cake on ceramic white plate.* [Image]. Unsplash. https://unsplash.com/photos/6SOc_IqY9mk

Cottonbro (2020). *Free elderly woman eating food stock photo*. [Image].Pexels. https://www.pexels.com/photo/elderly-woman-eating-food-5962042/

Hansel, L. (2020). *Pink and white oblong ornament photo*. [Image].Unsplash. https://unsplash.com/photos/pKsgUVm6PC0

Hume, C. (2017). *Person using MacBook*. [Image]. Unsplash. https://unsplash.com/photos/hBuwVLcYTnA

Fakurian, F. (2021). *Blue and green peacock feather*. [Image]. Unsplash. https://unsplash.com/photos/58Z17lnVS4U

Huizinga, A. (2018). *Selective focus photography*. [Image]. Unsplash. https://unsplash.com/photos/RmzR87vTiYw

Johnson, M. (2020). *Diabetes*. [Image]. Unsplash. https://unsplash.com/photos/4qjxCUOc3iQ

Jordan, B. (2021). *Brown wooden blocks on white surface*. [Image].Unsplash. https://unsplash.com/photos/vFGKWON91Bc

Kalos Skincare (2020). *Woman in white bathrobe*. [Image]. Unsplash. https://unsplash.com/photos/jyKa0Ynxvow

Kinney, C. (2018). *Person holding black exercise rope*. [Image]. Unsplash. https://unsplash.com/photos/FMQBLyhD2HU

Marras, A. (2017). *Bowl of ramen photo*. [Image]. Unsplash. https://unsplash.com/photos/SdS_XZ2CBqo

Poepperl, S. (2021). *White and gold round ceramic plate photo*. [Image]. Unsplash. https://unsplash.com/photos/2GFKGjjHM

Rae, S. (2017). *Brown dried leaves on sand photo* [Image]. Unsplash. https://unsplash.com/photos/geM5lzDj4Iw

Reproductive Health Supplies Coalition (2019). *Oral contraceptive pill on blue panel.* [Image]. Unsplash. https://unsplash.com/photos/gRRtWpFFMK8

Silviarita (2018). *Woman dragon relax* [Image]. Pixabay. https://pixabay.com/photos/woman-dragon-relax-tame-fantasy-3613722/

Siora Photography (2018). *Selective focus photography of tape measure.* [Image]. Unsplash.https://unsplash.com/photos/cixohzDpNIo

Shvets, A. (2020). *Elderly woman looking at mirror* [Image]. Pexels.https://www.pexels.com/photo/elderly-woman-looking-at-mirror-5231290/

Tyrrell Fitness and Nutrition (2021). *Green broccoli on white ceramic plate.* [Image]. Unsplash. https://unsplash.com/photos/jSQxj-Ug0H8

Made in the USA
Las Vegas, NV
06 April 2023